MCQS IN SURGERY

MCQS IN SURGERY

C. P. SHEARMAN

BSc, MS, FRCS, Consultant Surgeon,
Southampton University Hospital Trust,
Southampton

N. C. HICKEY

MD, FRCS, Consultant Surgeon,
Worcester Royal Infirmary

BAILLIÈRE TINDALL
LONDON PHILADELPHIA TORONTO
SYDNEY TOKYO

Baillière Tindall
W. B. Saunders

24–28 Oval Road
London NW1 7DX, UK

The Curtis Center
Independence Square West
Philadelphia, PA 19106-3399
USA

Harcourt Brace & Company
55 Horner Avenue
Toronto, Ontario M8Z 4X6
Canada

Harcourt Brace & Company
Australia
30–52 Smidmore Street
Marrickville, NSW 2204
Australia

Harcourt Brace & Company
Japan
Ichibancho Central Building
22-1 Ichibancho
Chiyoda-ku, Tokyo 102, Japan

© 1994 Baillière Tindall

All rights reserved. No part of this publication may be reproduced, stored in a retrieval system or transmitted, in any form or by any means, electronic, mechanical, photocopying or otherwise, without the prior permission of Baillière Tindall, 24–28 Oval Road, London NW1 7DX, UK

A catalogue record for this book is available from the British Library

ISBN 0–7020–1761–2

This book is printed on acid-free paper

Typeset by Paston Press Ltd, Loddon, Norfolk
Printed in Great Britain by Mackays of Chatham PLC, Chatham, Kent

Contents

Preface	vii
Introduction	ix
Paper 1	**1**
Paper 2	**13**
Paper 3	**27**
Paper 4	**41**
Paper 5	**53**
Answers to paper 1	65
Answers to paper 2	93
Answers to paper 3	123
Answers to paper 4	151
Answers to paper 5	179
Index	**207**

PREFACE

A major part of medical student assessment is currently by multiple choice questions (MCQs). Though these can be useful in reflecting a student's level of knowledge reasonably objectively, they can also be confusing and exam candidates who have mastered the technique of approaching them correctly and gained an understanding of their nature can be at a considerable advantage. Also, MCQs can appear ambiguous and students may find difficulty in understanding why a particular answer is designated right or wrong by the examiner.

When we were asked to write a series of surgery MCQs to help students prepare for examinations, we felt it would be inappropriate merely to provide lists of questions with our 'correct' and 'incorrect' answers. Across as broad a range of subjects as possible we have therefore provided questions with answers backed up by brief explanations, plus concise overviews of each topic addressed. Thus, students should be able to test their level of knowledge and revise a wide range of topics while getting a feel for the nature of MCQs in general.

Throughout the book we have arranged questions in the apparently random order students might find in an exam. However, by referring to the index, readers will be able to select all questions on a particular subject, such as vascular surgery or orthopaedics. They will therefore be able to use the book for two different purposes. By working through each section of the book from front to back they will be able to identify those areas in which they perform badly and need to undertake further revision. By working through a single topic they will be able to test their knowledge, and revise that particular field.

Readers should note that explanations of answers are brief and are intended to act largely as 'aides memoires' within subject areas already studied. If the information given appears to be new and unfamiliar, more detailed study is required.

C. P. SHEARMAN
N. C. HICKEY

INTRODUCTION

This book consists of 250 multiple choice questions covering areas with which a medical student should be familiar by the time he or she has completed the clinical course. Subjects for questions include General and Vascular Surgery, ENT, Neurosurgery, Urology, Orthopaedics, Paediatric Surgery, Pain Relief and Anaesthesia.

Questions are arranged in blocks of 50 such that each block can be considered as a separate exam that should be completed in no more than 1 hour 30 minutes. Alternatively, by referring to the index and selecting the question numbers listed the student may choose instead to revise one of the particular surgical areas mentioned above, or a narrower topic.

Each question consists of a stem with five possible responses that must be designated true or false by the student. The answers selected can then be checked against the answers grouped at the back of the book. The following system should be followed for scoring: one mark awarded for a correct response, one mark deducted for an incorrect response, and no adjustment to the score if a question remains unanswered.

Each set of five answers is followed by a brief description of the topic that that question addressed. This is intended to refresh the reader's memory on that topic and simultaneously to illustrate why answers have been designated correct or incorrect. We hope this will allow students to gain insight into the construction of MCQs and to develop their strategy for these exams.

Paper 1

1. *Abdominal aortic aneurysms (AAA):*
   (a) Often cause back pain.
   (b) Are usually found on careful abdominal examination.
   (c) Are more common in the close relatives of those with AAAs.
   (d) Occur equally in both sexes.
   (e) Are more frequent in patients with intermittent claudication.

2. *Adenocarcinoma of the oesophagus:*
   (a) May be excluded as a cause of dysphagia by barium swallow examination.
   (b) Is the commonest tumour affecting the lower third of the oesophagus.
   (c) May be effectively palliated by radiotherapy.
   (d) May occur secondarily to achalasia.
   (e) Carries a poor prognosis.

3. *Coronary artery bypass grafting (CABG):*
   (a) Should not be performed in patients with severe angina.
   (b) May use the internal mammary artery (IMA) as a 'living' conduit.
   (c) Carries an in-hospital mortality of over 20%.
   (d) In the absence of long saphenous vein (LSV), a polytetrafluoroethylene (PTFE) prosthesis is a useful alternative.
   (e) Is now only performed if percutaneous angioplasty fails.

4. *The following have some predictive value in the assessment of the severity of acute pancreatitis:*
   (a) The total white-cell count (WCC).
   (b) Serum amylase level.

(c) Arterial oxygen saturation (P_aO_2).
(d) Ultrasonography.
(e) Serum calcium.

5. *Reflux oesophagitis:*
   (a) May present with dysphagia.
   (b) Is invariably associated with a hiatus hernia.
   (c) Is most effectively treated in the acute stage by H_2-receptor antagonists.
   (d) Is usually caused by bile reflux.
   (e) May be surgically corrected by fundoplication.

6. *Prolapse of an intervertebral disc:*
   (a) Cannot be visualized by magnetic resonance imaging (MRI).
   (b) Most commonly occurs in the lower thoracic spine.
   (c) Occurs equally in males and females.
   (d) At L4/5 can result in brisk knee jerks.
   (e) May precipitate urinary retention.

7. *Ureteric stones:*
   (a) Rarely cause haematuria.
   (b) Occur more commonly in females.
   (c) Should be removed if there is infection in the kidney above the stones.
   (d) Usually show on a plain abdominal X-ray.
   (e) Can sometimes be dissolved with oral penicillamine.

8. *Mammographic screening for breast cancer in the UK:*
   (a) Is useful in all women after menarche.
   (b) Must be performed every 6 months to be effective.
   (c) Has involved women between the ages of 50 and 64 years.
   (d) Has resulted in the removal of five benign lesions for every cancer found.
   (e) Has been performed by a single oblique view of each breast.

9. *Carpal tunnel syndrome:*
   (a) Is associated with pregnancy.
   (b) Usually presents with weakness of finger flexion.
   (c) May be confirmed by nerve conduction studies.
   (d) Produces symptoms that are worse on use of the hand.
   (e) Can be treated by surgical decompression.

10. *Fractured neck of femur (NOF):*
    (a) Occurs most commonly in elderly females.
    (b) Presents with pain and a shortened, internally rotated leg.
    (c) Is best treated by early internal fixation.
    (d) Is associated with a 30-day mortality of about 30%.
    (e) Requires prolonged bed-rest.

11. *Duodenal ulcers:*
    (a) Should be routinely biopsied to exclude malignancy.
    (b) Are increasing in incidence.
    (c) May be associated with gastric colonization with *Helicobacter pylori*.
    (d) Are unlikely to recur after a course of H_2-receptor antagonists.
    (e) Are usually associated with gastric acid hypersecretion.

12. *Patients with intermittent claudication due to an atheromatous occlusion of the superficial femoral artery:*
    (a) Usually get worse if untreated.
    (b) May be treated by transluminal angioplasty.
    (c) Should have an angiogram to confirm the diagnosis.
    (d) May be treated by chemical sympathectomy.
    (e) Are very likely to have ischaemic heart disease.

13. *Inguinal hernias:*
    (a) Are usually direct when found in young men.
    (b) Are effectively controlled by a truss in patients unfit for surgery.
    (c) Should be repaired with absorbable sutures to avoid infection and fistulas.
    (d) May be repaired under local anaesthetic.
    (e) After repair, bed-rest should be advised for 5 days.

14. *Non-toxic nodular goitre (NTNG):*
    (a) Occurs as a result of iodine deficiency.
    (b) May cause tracheal compression.
    (c) Is associated with raised serum thyroxine levels.
    (d) Usually regresses spontaneously.
    (e) Should always be excised for fear of malignant change.

15. *Concerning pain relief after major abdominal surgery:*
    (a) Local anaesthetic infiltration is unhelpful.
    (b) Pethidine is effective, 4-hourly intramuscularly.
    (c) Non-steroidal anti-inflammatory drugs may reduce the pain.
    (d) Moderately severe pain is unavoidable in the first 24 hours.
    (e) Oral slow-release morphine is effective.

16. *The risk of developing a malignant melanoma:*
    (a) Is highest in childhood.
    (b) Is increased in someone with numerous moles.
    (c) Is increased in someone with a history of repeated sunburn.
    (d) Is high in native Africans living in the tropics.
    (e) Is increased by smoking.

17. *Hydrocephalus:*
    (a) May follow an attack of meningitis.
    (b) May retard head growth in a young child due to the increased intracranial pressure.
    (c) In adults is commonly benign.
    (d) May be relieved by draining the cerebrospinal fluid (CSF) into the peritoneum.
    (e) May result in abnormal skull radiographs.

18. *In young women with an 'acute abdomen':*
    (a) Pain relief should not be administered until the surgeon has seen the patient.
    (b) Laparoscopy may be helpful.
    (c) Appendicitis is the most likely cause.
    (d) Abdominal X-ray is rarely helpful.
    (e) A positive Rovsing's sign excludes pelvic pathology.

19. *Seminoma of the testicle:*
    (a) Is an uncommon malignancy in young men.
    (b) Always presents with a testicular mass.
    (c) Has not usually metastasized at presentation.
    (d) Metastasizes to the inguinal lymph nodes.
    (e) Is radiosensitive.

20. *Tumours of the pharynx:*
    (a) May present with hoarseness of the voice.
    (b) Rarely spread to the regional lymph nodes.
    (c) May be associated with smoking.
    (d) Are generally treated by local excision of the tumour.
    (e) Are most often squamous cell carcinomas.

21. *A stenosis of the left internal carotid artery (ICA):*
    (a) Is an indication for a left carotid endarterectomy.
    (b) May cause a hemiparesis affecting the right arm and leg.
    (c) Can cause amaurosis fugax.
    (d) Will be associated with a bruit, audible on the left side of the neck.
    (e) Is likely to be due to fibromuscular hyperplasia due to turbulence of the carotid bifurcation.

22. *Wound infection after abdominal surgery:*
    (a) Increases the risk of dehiscence or herniation.
    (b) Usually results from contamination by airborne bacteria.
    (c) Is best prevented by seven days of antibiotics post-operatively.
    (d) When established, requires drainage.
    (e) May be effectively prevented by locally applied antibiotics or antiseptics.

23. *Ischaemic ulcers:*
    (a) Most commonly occur on the anterior aspect of the leg.
    (b) Can be treated with bed-rest and elevation.
    (c) Are treated by local excision and skin grafting.
    (d) Are painful.
    (e) Are common in patients with intermittent claudication.

24. *Concerning the management of a solitary thyroid nodule:*
    (a) Fine needle aspiration (FNA) cytology may assist in diagnosis.
    (b) Ultrasound scanning may reveal a cyst.
    (c) Malignant nodules are revealed as a 'hot-spot' on radioisotope scanning.
    (d) Should be very conservative as malignancy is rare.
    (e) Follicular adenomas require total thyroidectomy.

25. *Concerning patients who have suffered a subarachnoid haemorrhage (SAH):*
    (a) Rupture of an intracranial aneurysm is the commonest cause.
    (b) Most who survive the initial event recover completely.
    (c) Angiography should be undertaken immediately.
    (d) Headache and vomiting are common.
    (e) Level of consciousness is rarely impaired.

26. *Treatment of squamous cell carcinoma of the lung:*
    (a) Is ideally surgical.
    (b) Should be surgical when mediastinal lymph nodes are extensively involved.
    (c) Should usually be by chemotherapy rather than radiotherapy.
    (d) Is usually palliative.
    (e) Is more effective for central than for peripheral tumours.

27. *Fractures of the neck and proximal shaft of femur:*
    (a) May be usefully classified as intracapsular or extracapsular.
    (b) Displaced intracapsular fractures may require femoral head replacement.
    (c) Subtrochanteric fractures are frequently complicated by avascular necrosis of the femoral head.
    (d) Intracapsular fractures usually require open reduction before fixation.
    (e) May require total hip replacement.

28. *Carcinoma of the prostate:*
    (a) Can usually be diagnosed on rectal examination. F
    (b) Is associated with previous vasectomy. T
    (c) May be diagnosed by transrectal ultrasonography. F
    (d) Responds to phenoxybenzamine. F
    (e) Is treated by radical prostatectomy. F

29. *In the management of severe acute pancreatitis:*
    (a) Fluids should be given sparingly as pulmonary oedema is a likely complication. F
    (b) Proteolytic enzyme inhibitors reduce the mortality. F
    (c) Regular arterial blood gas estimations should be performed. T
    (d) An ultrasound scan may be useful. T
    (e) Surgery has no place. F

30. *A patient presenting with haematuria:*
    (a) May have renal tract calculi. T
    (b) If no cause is found after investigation the patient can be discharged. F
    (c) In whom intravenous urogram (IVU) or ultrasound is normal then cystoscopy does not need to be performed. F
    (d) May have a urinary-tract infection. T
    (e) Should only be investigated if bleeding persists or it is the second episode. F

31. *Following Colles fracture of the wrist:*
    (a) X-rays reveal dorsal displacement and angulation with impaction of the distal radius. T
    (b) Ulnar nerve damage is common. F
    (c) Internal fixation is usually the treatment of choice. F
    (d) Malunion frequently occurs. T
    (e) Closed manipulation is usually appropriate. T

32. *The following are characteristics of carcinomas:*
    (a) They usually originate from connective tissue. F
    (b) Local invasion of surrounding tissues occurs. T
    (c) Early blood-borne metastases are likely. F

(d) An irregular mass, which may be ulcerated.
(e) A false capsule.

33. *Scoliosis of the spine:*
    (a) May be associated with hip deformity.
    (b) Is most commonly due to spina bifida.
    (c) Intervention should be started in childhood.
    (d) Cannot be corrected surgically.
    (e) May cause recurrent chest infections.

34. *In a patient suspected of having a perforated peptic ulcer:*
    (a) If there is no free gas visible on the erect chest X-ray the diagnosis is unlikely.
    (b) The ulcer is most likely to be situated on the lesser curvature of the stomach.
    (c) If the patient is taking non-steroidal anti-inflammatory drugs (NSAIDs) vagotomy should be performed to prevent recurrence.
    (d) Mortality is related to the time from perforation to treatment.
    (e) Simple closure with an omental patch gives an unacceptable ulcer recurrence rate and should be avoided.

35. *Epidural anaesthesia:*
    (a) May be preferable to general anaesthesia in patients undergoing femoropopliteal bypass grafting.
    (b) Is particularly useful in patients with chronic obstructive airways disease (COAD).
    (c) Is safer than general anaesthesia in patients with coronary artery disease and aortic valve stenosis.
    (d) Produces peripheral lower limb vasoconstriction.
    (e) Is contraindicated in anticoagulated patients.

36. *In a patient presenting with an acutely ischaemic leg:*
    (a) Neurosensory deficit is an indication for urgent intervention.
    (b) Angiography is rarely helpful.
    (c) Intravenous streptokinase should be given as a bolus.

(d) Many patients have a preceding history of symptoms of leg ischaemia.
(e) Elevation of the leg often reduces the pain.

37. *Following a major burn injury:*
    (a) Fluid requirements are greatest within the first 2 hours of injury.
    (b) Pulmonary oedema can occur even if the lung has not been injured.
    (c) Pain is initially worse in the less severely burnt areas.
    (d) Prophylactic antibiotics may be given on admission.
    (e) Intravenous H_2-receptor antagonists are usually given.

38. *Arteriovenous fistulas:*
    (a) Usually close spontaneously with time.
    (b) May follow a penetrating injury such as a stab wound.
    (c) Can result in heart failure.
    (d) Do not cause ischaemia.
    (e) May be treated by embolization.

39. *Crush fractures of the lumbar vertebrae:*
    (a) Commonly occur in road traffic accidents due to rapid deceleration.
    (b) Need surgical reduction and fixation.
    (c) Often occur after a fall from a height.
    (d) May be pathological.
    (e) Usually cause paraplegia.

40. *The prognosis of a malignant melanoma:*
    (a) Is better for a nodular than for a superficial spreading melanoma.
    (b) Is unaffected by clinical stage at presentation.
    (c) Is excellent for a melanoma less than 0.76 mm thick.
    (d) Is related to the level of histological invasion.
    (e) Is better for a limb lesion than for a trunk primary.

41. *Papillary carcinoma of the thyroid:*
    (a) Usually occurs in the first three decades.
    (b) Is characterized by early blood-borne dissemination to bone.

(c) Should be treated by radiotherapy.
(d) Is effectively treated by thyroidectomy followed by oral thyroxine replacement.
(e) Has a very poor prognosis.

42. *Deep vein thrombosis (DVT) in patients undergoing surgery:*
    (a) Occurs in less than 5% of patients undergoing abdominal operations.
    (b) Begins to form in the early post-operative period.
    (c) May lead to venous ulceration.
    (d) Is usually of little clinical significance.
    (e) Can be diagnosed with duplex ultrasound.

43. *Following a fracture dislocation of the spine between T10 and L1:*
    (a) Initial complete motor paralysis of the legs may completely recover.
    (b) If the patient is paraplegic urgent surgical decompression of the spinal cord must be undertaken.
    (c) Treatment is analgesia and early mobilization.
    (d) Persistent sensory loss in the legs with a normal anal reflex suggests cord transection.
    (e) Urinary retention may occur without the patient being aware.

44. *Fractured ribs:*
    (a) Should be treated by adhesive strapping to the chest wall.
    (b) Are readily diagnosed on a chest X-ray.
    (c) May be complicated by pneumothorax.
    (d) Invariably require the patient to be admitted to hospital.
    (e) Are especially dangerous if the first rib is broken.

45. *Rheumatoid arthritis (RA) of the cervical spine:*
    (a) Is common in patients with RA in other joints.
    (b) May cause instability of the atlantoaxial joint.
    (c) Should be identified before undertaking a general anaesthetic.

(d) Cannot be helped surgically.
(e) May be adequately treated with a cervical collar.

46. *Following a kick in the loin of a fit young man:*
    (a) Haematuria is an indication for surgical exploration of the kidney.
    (b) An intravenous urogram (IVU) should be obtained.
    (c) An angiogram is indicated if there is evidence that bleeding is continuing.
    (d) Bleeding may occur a week or so after the initial injury.
    (e) A damaged ureter is the most likely cause of haematuria.

47. *In patients in whom the diagnosis of acute appendicitis is suspected:*
    (a) The neutrophil count is often normal in appendicitis.
    (b) The development of an appendix mass is an indication for urgent surgical intervention.
    (c) An abdominal X-ray will show gas in the distended appendix lumen.
    (d) Ultrasound may be diagnostic.
    (e) Leucocytes in the urine exclude the diagnosis.

48. *Ischaemic rest pain of the lower limb:*
    (a) Implies imminent limb loss and is an indication for amputation.
    (b) Is worse in the thigh due to the large bulk of muscle.
    (c) Is usually worse at night.
    (d) Is most commonly due to small blood vessel disease in the foot and is not amenable to surgical bypass.
    (e) Should be treated by lumbar sympathectomy.

49. *Achalasia of the oesophagus:*
    (a) Usually presents with retrosternal pain.
    (b) Is associated with an increased risk of malignancy.
    (c) Is due to stricture formation at the cardia.
    (d) Occurs early in childhood.
    (e) Can be treated by balloon dilatation.

50. *Dislocation of the shoulder in a young adult:*
    (a) Most commonly follows a direct blow on the anterior aspect of the shoulder.
    (b) Reduced sensation over the deltoid suggests injury to the circumflex nerve.
    (c) Lateral X-rays may be helpful.
    (d) Recurrent dislocation usually requires surgical repair of the shoulder.
    (e) Following reduction the patient must be encouraged to begin using the arm to prevent muscle wasting.

Paper 2

1. *Adenocarcinoma of the kidney:*
   (a) Often presents with pain.
   (b) Rarely causes haematuria except in advanced cases.
   (c) Is treated by nephrectomy.
   (d) Should be treated with radiotherapy.
   (e) May invade the renal vein and inferior vena cava.

2. *Vesicoureteric reflux of urine:*
   (a) Is found in about one-third of children with bacteriuria.
   (b) Usually requires surgical reimplantation of the ureters to prevent permanent renal scarring.
   (c) Is best demonstrated by a micturating cystogram.
   (d) Should not be treated by long-term antibiotic prophylaxis as resistance is a problem.
   (e) May often resolve spontaneously.

3. *The prognosis for survival following treatment for breast cancer involving the axillary lymph nodes:*
   (a) Is related to the number of nodes found to be involved.
   (b) Is improved by adjuvant cytotoxic chemotherapy in women over 50 years of age.
   (c) Is improved by tamoxifen, especially in women over 50 years of age.
   (d) Is better following radical mastectomy than after local excision.
   (e) Is improved by local radiotherapy.

4. *Hirschsprung's disease:*
   (a) Is usually treated with laxatives.
   (b) Presents with absolute constipation within the first weeks of life.
   (c) Is due to abnormal ganglion cells in the rectum.
   (d) Is diagnosed on a full-thickness rectal biopsy.
   (e) Is associated with an absent rectosphincteric reflex.

5. *Pancreatic carcinoma:*
   (a) Is usually squamous-cell in origin.
   (b) Is increasing in incidence.
   (c) Is associated with a 5-year survival of 50%.
   (d) Is readily diagnosed by ultrasound scanning.
   (e) Is associated with diabetes mellitus.

6. *Supracondylar fracture of the humerus:*
   (a) May cause ischaemia of the arm.
   (b) Open reduction is the optimum treatment.
   (c) After reduction the elbow is kept flexed until union has occurred.
   (d) Is most common in children.
   (e) Remodelling occurs at the fracture site which will correct any residual deformity.

7. *Cancer of the tongue:*
   (a) Commonly metastasizes to local lymph nodes.
   (b) May arise in areas of leucoplakia.
   (c) Is usually treated by surgical resection.
   (d) Carries a better prognosis if arising from the posterior part of the tongue.
   (e) Is an adenocarcinoma and does not respond to radiotherapy.

8. *In a healthy 70-kg man:*
   (a) 60% of the body weight is water.
   (b) Circulating blood volume is 12 litres.
   (c) Intracellular fluid contains 4–4.5 mmol/l of potassium.
   (d) The predominant anion of extracellular fluid is chloride.
   (e) There is a negligible amount of interstitial fluid.

9. *Atheromatous stenosis of a renal artery:*
   (a) Is a cause of hypertension.
   (b) Does not impair renal function.
   (c) Can be treated by percutaneous, transluminal angioplasty.
   (d) May produce an audible bruit.

(e) Requiring surgical intervention necessitates nephrectomy.

10. *It has been demonstrated that post-operative deep vein thromboses (DVT) can be reduced by:*
    (a) Low dose aspirin.
    (b) Compression stockings.
    (c) Subcutaneous heparin on induction of anaesthesia.
    (d) Keeping operating times to a minimum.
    (e) Stopping the contraceptive pill (low-dose oestrogen) 6 weeks prior to surgery.

11. *A subdural empyema:*
    (a) May originate from a paranasal sinus infection.
    (b) Should be treated with steroids.
    (c) May require craniectomy.
    (d) Is often confirmed as the diagnosis by computerized tomography (CT) scanning.
    (e) Often follows a subarachnoid haemorrhage.

12. *An inguinal hernia in a child:*
    (a) Is associated with a patent processus vaginalis.
    (b) Should only be diagnosed after demonstrating the hernia on coughing.
    (c) Should not be operated on until the age of 5 years, as spontaneous closure may occur.
    (d) If irreducible, requires an emergency operation.
    (e) Is treated by simple inguinal herniotomy.

13. *Fibroadenomas of the breast:*
    (a) Should always be removed due to risk of malignant change.
    (b) Classically occur as a well-defined mobile lump in a young woman.
    (c) When diagnosed clinically, should be confirmed by mammography.
    (d) Occur most commonly in the upper, outer breast quadrant.
    (e) Are usually painful.

14. *Fractures of mandible:*
    (a) Are invariably compound and antibiotics should be given.
    (b) Are more common in elderly edentulous patients.
    (c) Are often missed due to facial swelling and bruising.
    (d) Areas of numbness under the lower lip suggest a fracture has occurred.
    (e) Treatment is generally conservative.

15. *Anal carcinomas:*
    (a) Should be treated by abdominoperineal excision of the anus and rectum.
    (b) Do not respond to radiotherapy.
    (c) May metastasize to the inguinal lymph nodes.
    (d) Are associated with the human papilloma virus.
    (e) May present with intestinal obstruction.

16. *Acute sinusitis:*
    (a) Can be diagnosed on X-ray.
    (b) Requires surgical drainage.
    (c) May cause a brain abscess.
    (d) Can follow a dental abscess.
    (e) Is most commonly viral and does not respond to antibiotics.

17. *Lipomas:*
    (a) Are confined to the subcutaneous fat.
    (b) May exhibit a sense of fluctuation on examination.
    (c) Should be excised for fear of malignant change.
    (d) May be treated by aspiration.
    (e) Are usually lobulated and encapsulated.

18. *In the control of water and sodium metabolism:*
    (a) Antidiuretic hormone (ADH) is released from the anterior lobe of the pituitary gland.
    (b) ADH increases the permeability of the distal convoluted tubules in the kidney to water.
    (c) ADH is released only on stimulation of the osmoreceptors by hypertonicity of the plasma.

(d) Decreased circulating volume activates the renin–angiotensin system, which stimulates aldosterone secretion and results in decreased urinary sodium excretion.
(e) Daily extrarenal water loss is about 1 litre.

19. *When considering intravenous fluid replacement:*
    (a) 5% dextrose is an important source of calories to the catabolic post-operative patient.
    (b) Normal saline contains 0.8 mmol/l of sodium.
    (c) Normal saline contains a greater concentration of chloride ions than does plasma.
    (d) A healthy adult requires about 2.5 litres of fluid per day.
    (e) Volume should be reduced in pyrexial patients, as fluid overload is more likely.

20. *In a fit patient with simple varicose veins and no history of a deep vein thrombosis:*
    (a) Surgery should be undertaken to prevent the development of venous ulcers.
    (b) Venography must be undertaken prior to surgery to ensure the deep veins are patent.
    (c) Stripping of the long saphenous vein (LSV) from the groin to the ankle prevents recurrence of varicose veins.
    (d) Long saphenous incompetence (LSI) can be detected by simple clinical tests.
    (e) Short saphenous incompetence (SSI) must be excluded.

21. *Familial adenomatous polyposis coli (FAP):*
    (a) Is an autosomal dominant inherited condition.
    (b) Is always found to affect other family members if checked carefully.
    (c) Usually presents in childhood with rectal bleeding.
    (d) Carries a risk of malignant transformation of 10% over 10 years of age.
    (e) Is associated with retinal abnormalities.

22. *Carcinoma of the maxillary antrum:*
    (a) May present with toothache.
    (b) Should be treated by wide surgical excision.
    (c) Is not effectively staged by computerized tomography (CT) scanning of the head.
    (d) May cause symptoms suggestive of sinusitis.
    (e) Is rarely radiosensitive.

23. *Venous ulcers:*
    (a) May be treated by elevation and compression.
    (b) Are due to capillary stasis.
    (c) Rarely heal without surgical intervention.
    (d) Occur at the sites of varicose veins.
    (e) Are usually infected and should be treated with topical antibiotics.

24. *Patients with osteoarthritis of the hip:*
    (a) May present with pain in the knee.
    (b) May benefit from femoral osteotomy.
    (c) Have wide joint spaces on X-ray due to bony destruction.
    (d) Rarely suffer pain when resting at night.
    (e) Suffer joint stiffness and pain that is often worse in the morning.

25. *In a patient who has recently passed a renal stone:*
    (a) Serum calcium should be measured when the patient has fully recovered.
    (b) Long-term antibiotics are necessary to prevent recurrence.
    (c) An increase in fluid intake should be encouraged.
    (d) A 24-hour urine collection should be obtained.
    (e) An intravenous urogram should be obtained.

26. *Incompletely descended testicle:*
    (a) Is associated with testicular dysplasia.
    (b) Should be brought down to the scrotum before the age of 2 years to reduce the risk of malignancy.
    (c) May be palpated in the scrotum at birth, but the cord

fails to grow with the child and becomes incompletely descended later.
(d) Is differentiated from a retractile testicle by milking the latter into the scrotum, a procedure best performed with the child standing up.
(e) May sometimes remain intra-abdominal.

27. *Cyclical mastalgia:*
    (a) Is often worse just before menstruation.
    (b) Is usually associated with nodularity of the breasts.
    (c) Is frequently the presenting symptom of carcinoma.
    (d) May be due to abnormal essential fatty acid (EFA)/prostaglandin metabolism.
    (e) Is unaffected by hormone replacement therapy (HRT).

28. *Adenomatous polyps of the large bowel:*
    (a) Usually cause symptoms of bleeding.
    (b) Are often multiple.
    (c) After removal patients should be followed-up by regular colonoscopy.
    (d) Have a malignant potential that is proportional to their size.
    (e) May present with hypokalaemia.

29. *In a patient undergoing a total hip arthroplasty (THA):*
    (a) Prophylactic antibiotics should be given.
    (b) Loosening of the femoral component is a cause of pain.
    (c) Deep vein thrombosis (DVT) may occur in up to one-third of patients.
    (d) Rheumatoid arthritis is a contraindication for THA.
    (e) Dislocation of the prosthesis in the first few days is treated by surgical revision.

30. *In the treatment of varicose veins:*
    (a) Injection sclerotherapy is only of value for small, recurrent veins.
    (b) Deep venous reflux is often improved by sapheno-femoral vein ligation.
    (c) Graduated compression stockings are used only as a temporary measure.

(d) Failure to palpate ankle pulses in a patient with varicose veins is usually due to oedema of the limb.
(e) Small varicose veins may be avulsed through tiny 'stab' incisions.

31. *In the treatment of carcinoma of the head of the pancreas:*
    (a) Endoscopic stenting of an obstructed bile duct is only undertaken if the patient is unfit for surgery.
    (b) Radical surgery (pancreaticoduodenectomy) is associated with an increased survival and should usually be undertaken.
    (c) Carcinoembryonic antigen (CEA) is raised only if liver metastases are present.
    (d) Radiotherapy is a useful alternative to surgery for advanced tumours.
    (e) Coeliac axis block may help control pain.

32. *Pneumothorax:*
    (a) Presents with dyspnoea and chest pain with absent breath sounds and hyper-resonance on examination.
    (b) May require no treatment.
    (c) If of the tension (valvular) variety, should be treated by intercostal tube drainage only after confirmation of the diagnosis with a chest X-ray.
    (d) If recurrent, may be treated by thoracoscopic pleurodesis.
    (e) May complicate mechanical ventilation.

33. *A patient with diabetes undergoing major abdominal surgery:*
    (a) Is at greater risk of infection than is a non-diabetic.
    (b) If insulin dependent, normal insulin doses should be administered pre-, per- and post-operatively.
    (c) If tablet controlled, oral hypoglycaemics should be omitted on the morning of surgery.
    (d) Is at greater risk of developing a deep venous thrombosis (DVT).
    (e) Carries a higher mortality risk than in a non-diabetic.

34. *Following an attack of acute tonsillitis in a child:*
    (a) Pain on opening the mouth may indicate a peritonsillar abscess.
    (b) Tonsillectomy should be undertaken to prevent further attacks.
    (c) Persistent enlargement of the tonsils is an indication for tonsillectomy.
    (d) If tonsillectomy is planned it should be undertaken as soon as possible before the tonsil becomes scarred and fibrotic.
    (e) In the presence of a previous cleft palate repair, tonsillectomy should be avoided if possible.

35. *Local analgesic (anaesthetic) infiltration for minor surgery:*
    (a) Is best performed with bupivacaine as this drug has the lowest systemic toxicity.
    (b) To digits should include adrenaline to prevent systemic spread.
    (c) Is effective immediately.
    (d) Should be performed with the highest concentration of agent available.
    (e) May be augmented by the cautious use of intravenous diazepam.

36. *The following are recognized risk factors for colorectal cancer:*
    (a) Familial adenomatous polyposis coli (FAP).
    (b) Diverticular disease.
    (c) Family history of colorectal cancer.
    (d) Angiodysplasia.
    (e) Inflammatory bowel disease.

37. *In patients with diverticular disease of the colon:*
    (a) Bleeding associated with large bowel diverticula rarely settles spontaneously and requires surgical intervention.
    (b) Pneumaturia may develop as a complication.
    (c) There is an increased risk of carcinoma of the colon.

(d) It is likely that there are diverticula in the rest of the gastrointestinal tract.
(e) May present with large bowel obstruction.

38. *Metastatic carcinoma in bone:*
    (a) Is most likely to have arisen from the lung.
    (b) In men, is invariably osteolytic.
    (c) Is most effectively demonstrated by plain radiographs.
    (d) If leading to pathological fractures, should be treated by internal fixation.
    (e) Produces pain that may be relieved by radiotherapy.

39. *In a 50-year-old man with persistent hoarseness of the voice:*
    (a) Antibiotics should be commenced.
    (b) A chest X-ray should be obtained.
    (c) Indirect laryngoscopy is indicated.
    (d) Overuse of the voice is the most likely cause.
    (e) Pain in the ear suggests an upper-respiratory-tract infection as the most probable cause.

40. *Osteosarcomas:*
    (a) Most commonly present in the elderly.
    (b) Treatment is radiotherapy.
    (c) May be preceded by Paget's disease of the bone.
    (d) Lung metastases occur early.
    (e) May be mistaken for osteomyelitis.

41. *Paraoesophageal (rolling) hiatus hernias:*
    (a) Usually presents with symptoms of reflux oesophagitis.
    (b) Occur through a congenital diaphragmatic defect.
    (c) Is best diagnosed on barium meal examination.
    (d) Can usually be controlled with medical therapy.
    (e) May present with strangulation.

42. *Following a tear of the medial meniscus of the knee of a young man:*
    (a) Full extension of the knee is often not possible.
    (b) He will be at greater risk of secondary osteoarthritis in that knee.

(c) Underlying abnormalities of the meniscus are commonly found.
(d) A haemarthrosis generally occurs in the first hours of the injury.
(e) Arthroscopic examination of the knee may be needed to confirm the diagnosis.

43. *Septic shock syndrome:*
    (a) Is initially associated with a low central venous pressure (CVP).
    (b) Is characterized by cold, sweaty extremities.
    (c) Results in pulmonary oedema.
    (d) Should not be treated with antibiotics until bacterial sensitivities are known.
    (e) Commonly results from Gram-negative organisms from the biliary, gastrointestinal or urinary tracts.

44. *In a patient with an extensive post-operative deep vein thrombosis (DVT):*
    (a) Initial treatment should be intravenous heparin.
    (b) Prior to anticoagulation, intravenous streptokinase should be given to lyse the thrombus.
    (c) Heparin should be given, 5000 units subcutaneously, twice daily.
    (d) Oral anticoagulants are commenced when the clinical signs of the DVT have gone.
    (e) Heparin therapy is best determined on a units per kilogram body weight basis.

45. *In a seriously injured young male motorcyclist with a suspected fractured pelvis:*
    (a) Blood visible at the external meatus of the penis is suggestive of urethral injury.
    (b) No attempt should be made to catheterize the bladder to avoid possible injury to the urethra.
    (c) A catheter can usually be passed if a rigid introducer is used.
    (d) Suprapubic catheterization is often the best option.
    (e) Surgical repair of the urethra must be undertaken within the first few hours to avoid irreparable damage.

46. *A 12-year-old boy presenting with a short history of a limp and painful hip:*
    (a) Will most likely have a previously undiagnosed congenital dislocation of the hip (CDH).
    (b) Slipped femoral epiphysis must be considered.
    (c) If X-rays are normal, the boy should be encouraged to exercise to prevent joint stiffening.
    (d) If infection is suspected, aspiration of the hip joint must be carried out.
    (e) May have rheumatoid arthritis.

47. *In ulcerative colitis (UC):*
    (a) Fistulas frequently form between loops of bowel.
    (b) Barium enema may show pseudopolyps.
    (c) Orosomucoid is a specific disease activity marker.
    (d) Toxic dilatation of the colon requires urgent colectomy.
    (e) The disease commonly starts in the terminal ileum.

48. *Congenital dislocation of the hip (CDH) in a 6-week-old baby:*
    (a) Should be diagnosed by routine X-ray of the hip.
    (b) May be suggested by the appearance of the groin skin creases.
    (c) Usually results in hip abduction being greater than normal.
    (d) Is more likely if a sibling has suffered from CDH.
    (e) Should be treated by splintage before the baby begins to crawl.

49. *Discharge from the nipple:*
    (a) In a woman of 65 years of age is very unlikely to be due to cancer.
    (b) If bloodstained, is invariably due to cancer.
    (c) When coloured (e.g. green) and opalescent is likely to be due to duct ectasia.
    (d) If milky (galactorrhoea), investigations should include a serum prolactin estimation.

(e) When associated with a breast lump, discharge should be controlled before considering investigation and treatment of the lump.

50. *A child with an atrial septal defect (ostium secundum):*
    (a) Usually presents with heart failure soon after birth.
    (b) Is cyanosed.
    (c) May present with recurrent chest infections.
    (d) On examination, usually demonstrates a murmur with fixed splitting of the second heart sound.
    (e) Requires surgical closure if the defect produces significantly increased pulmonary flow.

Paper 3

1. *In a patient with a proven, extensive deep vein thrombosis (DVT):*
   (a) Anticoagulation should be continued for at least 3 months.
   (b) A filter should be placed in the inferior vena cava to prevent a fatal pulmonary embolus.
   (c) Immediate surgical thrombectomy reduces the risk of pulmonary embolus and the subsequent development of chronic venous insufficiency.
   (d) Graduated compression stockings are usually prescribed.
   (e) If pregnant, prolonged heparin anticoagulation is usually undertaken.

2. *In acute hypovolaemic shock:*
   (a) A falling blood pressure is the most sensitive indicator.
   (b) Urine output is 1–2 ml/kg per hour.
   (c) Central venous pressure measurement provides a useful method of monitoring fluid replacement.
   (d) Peripheral vasodilatation occurs.
   (e) Respiratory rate falls.

3. *Primary thyrotoxicosis (Grave's disease):*
   (a) Is associated with ischaemia of the thyroid gland.
   (b) Is an autoimmune disease associated with increased levels of immunoglobulin G (IgG).
   (c) Should not be treated surgically due to the risk of thyrotoxic crisis post-operatively.
   (d) May be controlled by radio-iodine.
   (e) Must be treated by total thyroidectomy.

4. *A ganglion:*
   (a) Is a solid tumour of subcutaneous connective tissue.
   (b) Is fluctuant on examination.

(c) Should be treated by bursting by direct force.
(d) May be treated by aspiration and steroid injection.
(e) Often recurs after surgical excision.

5. *Aortic valve replacement:*
   (a) Requires cardiopulmonary bypass.
   (b) Is performed via a left thoracotomy.
   (c) May be performed for aortic valve regurgitation.
   (d) Is sometimes performed with a porcine heterograft.
   (e) Usually requires long-term anticoagulation post-operatively.

6. *In Crohn's disease:*
   (a) There is a peak onset in 20–40 year olds.
   (b) The inflammatory process is limited to the mucosa.
   (c) Patients may develop erythema nodosum (EN).
   (d) At operation, diseased segments of bowel should always be removed.
   (e) If total colectomy has to be undertaken, then an ileostomy can be avoided by fashioning an ileoanal pouch.

7. *Acute prolapse of a lumbar intervertebral disc:*
   (a) Most commonly protrudes centrally into the spinal canal.
   (b) May be associated with reduced ankle jerk reflexes.
   (c) Often follows excessive bending or lifting.
   (d) May involve two levels.
   (e) Requires urgent surgical decompression.

8. *Hypospadias:*
   (a) Is acquired due to balanitis in the first few months of life.
   (b) Is associated with a hooded foreskin.
   (c) Should be treated by early circumcision followed by correction of the urethral deformity at school age.
   (d) May require no treatment.
   (e) Is very rare.

9. *Obstructive jaundice is characterized by:*
   (a) Bilirubinuria.
   (b) An absence of urobilinogen in the urine.
   (c) Dark, bile-stained stools.
   (d) Reduced absorption of clotting factors III, IV, VII and XI.
   (e) Dilated intrahepatic bile ducts.

10. *The insertion of a chest drain:*
    (a) For pneumothorax, should usually be a basal drain in the 8th/9th intercostal space.
    (b) Is usually performed using local anaesthetic.
    (c) Involves cutting the skin only, then insertion of the drain by firm pressure on a sharp trocar.
    (d) Should be performed just underneath a rib to avoid intercostal vessels and nerve.
    (e) Should be followed by connection to an underwater seal system.

11. *Prolonged severe vomiting may result in:*
    (a) Metabolic acidosis.
    (b) Hyperkalaemia.
    (c) Aciduria.
    (d) Cheyne–Stokes respiration.
    (e) Renal failure.

12. *In a patient suspected of having a deep vein thrombosis (DVT):*
    (a) The diagnosis should be confirmed using the iodine-125 fibrinogen uptake test.
    (b) Mobilization should be encouraged to prevent extension of the thrombus.
    (c) Duplex ultrasound may confirm the diagnosis.
    (d) They may not complain of any symptoms.
    (e) Clinical examination will confirm the diagnosis in the majority of cases.

13. *In a patient with a carcinoma of the colon:*
    (a) If the tumour is in the caecum, a right hemicolectomy is usually undertaken.

(b) If the lesion causes obstruction this should be relieved by the passage of a flatus tube.
(c) Post-operative radiotherapy improves survival.
(d) A very high carcinoembryonic antigen (CEA) is indicative of metastases.
(e) 3% of patients have more than one large bowel tumour at the time of presentation.

14. *A hydrocele in an elderly man:*
    (a) Is usually associated with an inguinal hernia.
    (b) Requires a testicular ultrasound scan to exclude malignancy.
    (c) Can be associated with heart failure.
    (d) May be treated by plicating the sac of the hydrocele with sutures.
    (e) Is unlikely to recur following simple aspiration.

15. *Portal hypertension:*
    (a) May result from hepatic vein thrombosis.
    (b) Causes hypersplenism.
    (c) Is complicated by the formation of haemorrhoids.
    (d) Is commonly complicated by ascites when due to portal vein thrombosis.
    (e) When complicated by oesophageal varices, may be treated by splenorenal shunting.

16. *Secretory otitis media:*
    (a) May present with conductive deafness.
    (b) Is a common cause of chronic ear discharge.
    (c) In an adult may be caused by a tumour.
    (d) May require surgical removal of the adenoids.
    (e) Is usually painful.

17. *Sudden pain and tenderness behind the knee in a 60-year-old man:*
    (a) Is unlikely to be a deep vein thrombosis (DVT) unless the man has recently had an operation.
    (b) May be a popliteal aneurysm.
    (c) If a swelling is present, it is a Baker's cyst which should be removed.

(d) Tears of the gastronemius muscle are unlikely unless the man has been involved in strenuous sport.
(e) Duplex ultrasound investigation is likely to be of value.

18. *In a young man, unconscious with a head injury following a road traffic accident:*
    (a) Extradural haematomas are the commonest cause of death.
    (b) Burr holes should be made immediately over the pterion of the skull.
    (c) Blood loss from the head injury itself is seldom significant.
    (d) Subarachnoid haemorrhage only occurs if there was an underlying abnormality.
    (e) A dilating pupil, unresponsive to light is a sign of increasing intracranial pressure.

19. *Basal cell carcinoma of the skin:*
    (a) Usually presents as a raised, pigmented lump on the upper body.
    (b) Metastasizes early to local lymph nodes.
    (c) Is pre-disposed to by exposure to sunlight.
    (d) May be treated effectively by surgical excision and grafting.
    (e) Is not radiosensitive.

20. *Gas gangrene:*
    (a) Is a common complication following amputation for peripheral vascular disease.
    (b) Results from mixed clostridial contamination, primarily by *Clostridium welchii*.
    (c) Is only diagnosed after crepitus is felt and gas is seen in the tissues on X-ray.
    (d) Is treated by resuscitation, antibiotics and surgical debridement.
    (e) Hyperbaric oxygen may be helpful.

21. *Carcinoma of the stomach:*
    (a) Is more likely to occur in patients with pernicious anaemia (PA).

(b) Is more likely to occur in patients with gastric hyperacidity.
(c) May present with anaemia and weight loss, without local symptoms.
(d) Spreads early via the blood stream to the ovaries.
(e) Carries a prognosis that is unrelated to the degree of spread at presentation.

22. *Osteoarthritis (OA) of the knee joint:*
    (a) Most commonly affects the femorotibial articulation.
    (b) Loose bodies may occur in the joint.
    (c) Arthrodesis is generally satisfactory treatment.
    (d) An effusion is present only during acute exacerbations of the condition.
    (e) Tibial osteotomy may relieve the symptoms.

23. *Strictures of the urethra:*
    (a) May be congenital in origin.
    (b) May follow transurethral resection of the prostate.
    (c) Should be treated by resection of the urethra and end-to-end anastomosis unless the stricture is short.
    (d) Can be diagnosed by urethrography.
    (e) May cause pneumaturia.

24. *Oesophageal atresia and tracheo-oesophageal fistula (TOF):*
    (a) Is associated with maternal hydramnios.
    (b) The usual deformity is the proximal oesophagus entering the trachea, with a blind distal oesophageal stump.
    (c) Presents with copious vomiting.
    (d) Requires urgent surgical intervention.
    (e) May be associated with cardiac and vertebral abnormalities.

25. *Pre-patellar bursitis:*
    (a) Is due to chronic inflammation of the bursa in front of the patella.
    (b) Is generally bacterial due to entry of organisms through broken skin.

(c) Surgical removal of the bursa is indicated if the condition is recurrent.
(d) Aspiration must not be performed as it may introduce infection.
(e) Is associated with osteoarthritis of the knee.

26. *Acute otitis media:*
    (a) May be relieved by myringotomy.
    (b) Requires grommets to be inserted to prevent recurrence.
    (c) Is usually viral.
    (d) May spontaneously resolve after rupture of the tympanic membrane.
    (e) May result in permanent deafness.

27. *When assessing the size and thickness of a major burn:*
    (a) Loss of pin-prick sensation suggests a full-thickness burn.
    (b) The area of a burn is of little clinical significance.
    (c) Scalds are more likely to produce full-thickness burns then are contact or flame burns.
    (d) The head and neck comprise about 9% of the adults surface area.
    (e) Hospital admission is only required for children when the burn size is estimated at >30% of the surface area.

28. *Accepted antibiotic prophylaxis for a patient undergoing elective large bowel surgery includes:*
    (a) No antibiotics.
    (b) A single intravenous dose of gentamicin and metronidazole given at the start of the operation.
    (c) Wound lavage with tetracycline.
    (d) Three perioperative doses of intravenous cefuroxime and metronidazole.
    (e) Three perioperative doses of intravenous flucloxacillin.

29. *Nasal polyps:*
    (a) May cause recurrent sinusitis.
    (b) May rarely be malignant.

(c) Are often associated with atopy and may improve with steroid sprays.
(d) Are associated with nasal discharge.
(e) Have a tendency to become malignant.

30. *Carcinoma of the stomach:*
    (a) Should be excluded by endoscopy in all patients over 40 years of age presenting with recent onset of dyspepsia.
    (b) Usually presents early, allowing the chance of cure by radical gastrectomy.
    (c) Adjuvant radiotherapy prolongs survival.
    (d) Cimetidine may reduce symptoms.
    (e) In the UK, has a 5-year survival rate of about 50%.

31. *In a patient undergoing infrarenal aortic aneurysm repair:*
    (a) In a male, impotence may occur post-operatively.
    (b) Adequate assessment of cardiac status can be obtained from the history and a clinical examination.
    (c) An angiogram should be obtained to determine the relationship of the renal arteries.
    (d) A computerized-tomography (CT) scan may distinguish an inflammatory aneurysm from a normal aneurysm.
    (e) Antibodies should be given prophylactically during the procedure.

32. *Day-case surgery:*
    (a) Has been made possible by the advent of laparoscopic surgery.
    (b) Is only suitable for procedures performed under local anaesthetic.
    (c) Should only be performed on patients who have easy access to a telephone.
    (d) Is especially useful for mobile independent patients who can drive home.
    (e) Is unsuitable for children.

33. *In a man presenting with acute retention of urine:*
    (a) Narcotic analgesia should be given to relieve the pain.
    (b) Suprapubic catheters may be used.
    (c) If it is not possible to pass a urethral catheter, an open prostatectomy will be required.
    (d) A transurethral resection of the prostate (TURP) will always be required.
    (e) An indwelling catheter can be left for as long as required without risk until surgical treatment is undertaken.

34. *Tennis elbow:*
    (a) There is localized pain over the lateral epicondyle.
    (b) Passive extension of the fingers causes pain.
    (c) Local steroid injection may help.
    (d) The radial nerve may be involved.
    (e) Surgery is of no value.

35. *In an elderly man with chronic urinary retention:*
    (a) Severe pain is not usually the presenting symptom.
    (b) A catheter should not be passed if the urine is infected.
    (c) Renal failure may develop.
    (d) A diuresis may develop if catheterized.
    (e) Transitional cell bladder tumours are a commonly associated finding.

36. *Concerning the management of a baby with suspected infantile hypertrophic pyloric stenosis:*
    (a) The diagnosis is confirmed by feeling a pyloric 'tumour' whilst the baby is feeding.
    (b) The baby is likely to be acidotic.
    (c) As soon as the diagnosis is confirmed, emergency pyloromyotomy is performed.
    (d) Oral feeding can be recommenced a few hours after surgery.
    (e) The condition presents most commonly in boys aged 4–6 weeks.

37. *Acute aortic dissection:*
    (a) Is more common in hypertensives.
    (b) Involves the stripping away of the intima from the rest of the aortic wall.
    (c) May present with acute lower limb ischaemia.
    (d) Resuscitation should involve control of blood pressure with intravenous hypotensive agents.
    (e) Involving the ascending aorta, is usually best treated surgically.

38. *Acute cholecystitis:*
    (a) May occur in the absence of gallstones.
    (b) Is usually associated with a normal white cell count.
    (c) Is characterized by an intolerance to fatty foods.
    (d) Should usually be treated by resuscitation, antibiotics and cholecystectomy.
    (e) May be associated with a raised serum amylase.

39. *In a patient with symptoms of Raynaud's phenomenon of the hands:*
    (a) There is usually an associated underlying connective tissue disorder.
    (b) Treatment with vasodilators is generally effective.
    (c) The diagnosis may be supported by infrared thermography.
    (d) Digital ulceration may occur.
    (e) There may be an underlying malignancy.

40. *A fistula connecting the jejunum to the abdominal skin:*
    (a) Is most commonly produced by perforation of a jejunal carcinoma.
    (b) Should be treated initially by an absorbent dressing and antibiotics.
    (c) Is unlikely to heal without surgical intervention.
    (d) Requires increased oral fluids and nutrition to promote healing.
    (e) Causes fluid and electrolyte depletion.

41. *Surgical cervical (dorsal) sympathectomy for upper limb problems:*
    (a) Is good first-line treatment for patients with Raynaud's phenomenon.
    (b) Gives good results for hyperhydrosis of the hands.
    (c) May be carried out thoracoscopically.
    (d) Horner's syndrome is a recognized complication.
    (e) Involves removing or destroying the sympathetic chain in the neck.

42. *Massive transfusion of stored blood risks:*
    (a) Impaired supply of oxygen to tissues.
    (b) Hypercalcaemia.
    (c) Myocardial impairment.
    (d) Adult respiratory disease syndrome (ARDS).
    (e) Hypercoagulability.

43. *Phaeochromocytoma:*
    (a) May be familial.
    (b) Is usually bilateral.
    (c) Frequently arises at a site distant from the adrenal glands.
    (d) Is associated with increased urinary vanillylmandelic acid (UMA).
    (e) May be localized by computerized tomography (CT) scanning.

44. *Sebaceous cysts:*
    (a) May occur on the palm of the hand.
    (b) May have a keratin-filled punctum at their centre.
    (c) Are easily moved under the skin.
    (d) May be multiple.
    (e) Are effectively treated by simple incision and drainage of the contents.

45. *In a young man with a deep laceration of the anterior aspect of the wrist after falling through a glass window:*
    (a) If there is a full function of the hand, simple primary suture should be performed.

(b) Flexor tendon injury should be repaired by primary suture if the wound is clean.
(c) A tourniquet should be used if surgical exploration of the wound is required.
(d) X-rays of the area should be obtained.
(e) Repair of the wound should be carried out under general anaesthesia.

46. *Concerning tumours of the larynx:*
    (a) They may present with stridor.
    (b) They may be diagnosed by laryngoscopy.
    (c) If malignant, rarely arise on the true cord.
    (d) Benign polyps are the commonest cause of hoarseness.
    (e) Hyperkeratosis is sometimes found on the cord.

47. *Following splenectomy:*
    (a) The platelet count usually rises.
    (b) There is an increased risk of *Haemophilus influenzae* infections.
    (c) The increased risk of pneumococcal infections can be greatly reduced by pneumococcal vaccine given 6 weeks post-operatively.
    (d) Children are not at increased risk of infection.
    (e) The earliest sign of increased susceptibility to infection is subphrenic abscess post-operatively.

48. *In a patient who is acutely unwell with severe abdominal pain:*
    (a) An erect chest X-ray may be useful.
    (b) A serum amylase is unlikely to be useful unless gallstones are seen on an ultrasound scan.
    (c) A white cell count of $30 \times 10^9/l$ suggests acute appendicitis.
    (d) The presence of rebound tenderness is sought by pressing firmly on the abdomen, suddenly releasing the fingers and asking the patient if the pain increased on release.
    (e) Guarding suggests peritonitis.

49. *Rheumatoid arthritis affecting the hand:*
    (a) Spontaneous rupture of the tendons may occur.
    (b) The distal interphalangeal joints (DIPJ) are most commonly involved.
    (c) The fingers tend to deviate to the ulnar side.
    (d) Splintage of affected joints may reduce pain.
    (e) Serum rheumatoid factor is positive.

50. *Features suggesting appendicitis rather than mesenteric adenitis as a cause of an acute abdomen in a child include:*
    (a) Temperature greater than 38°C.
    (b) Cervical adenitis.
    (c) Guarding.
    (d) Rebound tenderness.
    (e) Headache.

Paper 4

1. *Primary treatment of invasive ductal carcinoma of the breast in a 60-year-old woman:*
   (a) Requires mastectomy.
   (b) Should include surgical excision of axillary lymph nodes followed by radiotherapy.
   (c) May be by local excision and adjuvant radiotherapy.
   (d) Should routinely include adjuvant tamoxifen.
   (e) Should routinely include adjuvant chemotherapy.

2. *Prostatitis:*
   (a) Can be sexually transmitted.
   (b) Should be treated by antibiotics for at least 6 weeks.
   (c) May result in a prostatic abscess.
   (d) May follow urethral catheterization.
   (e) May follow urethroscopy.

3. *Dupuytren's contracture:*
   (a) Is due to fibrous shortening of the flexor tendons of the ring and little fingers.
   (b) May require amputation of the affected digit.
   (c) Steroid injections into the affected area are effective treatment.
   (d) Excision of the fibrous tissue can improve the situation considerably.
   (e) The condition is often bilateral.

4. *Testicular teratomas:*
   (a) Most commonly occur between the ages of 20 and 30 years.
   (b) Are germ cell tumours originating from a totipotential embryonal cell.
   (c) Spread via lymphatics to the inguinal lymph nodes.

(d) May provoke an increase in serum alpha-fetoprotein and human chorionic gonadotrophin levels.
(e) Carry a poor prognosis.

5. *Intraperitoneal adhesions:*
   (a) Are invariably caused by starch from surgeons' gloves.
   (b) Result from peritoneal trauma, ischaemia or infection.
   (c) Once formed, are very likely to cause intestinal obstruction.
   (d) Are prevented by perioperative parenteral antibiotics.
   (e) May be reduced by careful surgical technique and peritoneal lavage.

6. *Patients who have sustained major burns:*
   (a) Require vigorous fluid replacement, especially 24–72 hours after the burn injury.
   (b) Have increased susceptibility to infection.
   (c) Develop negative nitrogen balance.
   (d) Rarely require blood transfusion.
   (e) Should be subjected to early aggressive oral rehydration therapy.

7. *The sudden development of stridor in a previously fit 5-year-old child:*
   (a) Is often the first presentation of asthma.
   (b) May diminish if the child's position is altered.
   (c) May be caused by infection.
   (d) Is an indication for emergency tracheostomy.
   (e) Is an indication for a chest X-ray to be obtained.

8. *Patients with thoracic outlet syndrome:*
   (a) May benefit from first rib resection.
   (b) Always have a cervical rib on X-ray.
   (c) May lose their radial pulse when their arm is externally rotated and abducted.
   (d) May present with subclavian vein thrombosis.
   (e) May present with acute ischaemia of the arm.

9. *In a man with an enlarged prostate gland:*
   (a) Symptoms are related to the size of the gland.
   (b) There is an increased risk of urinary-tract infection.

(c) Incontinence may result.
(d) Stilboestrol will reduce the symptoms.
(e) Chronic renal failure may occur.

10. *In a patient with a suspected fracture of the scaphoid bone:*
    (a) If no fracture is seen on X-ray the patient should be X-rayed again 2 weeks before applying a plaster cast.
    (b) Avascular necrosis is a particular concern.
    (c) The patient should be treated in a plaster cast that includes the thumb.
    (d) Osteoarthritis of the wrist may develop.
    (e) Primary internal fixation should be undertaken if the patient is a young manual worker.

11. *In a patient with severe epistaxis:*
    (a) A post-nasal pack should be inserted initially.
    (b) The patient should be sedated and placed supine in bed.
    (c) Bleeding commonly arises from the nasal septum.
    (d) A clotting screen should be undertaken if bleeding persists.
    (e) The patient should be nursed head down to protect the airway.

12. *Portwine stains of the skin:*
    (a) Tend to fade with time.
    (b) Are arteriovenous fistulas.
    (c) Should be treated by wide excision and skin grafting.
    (d) May be shrunk by laser therapy.
    (e) Only appear in adolescence.

13. *Peripheral nerve (PN) injuries:*
    (a) Common peroneal nerve injury causes foot drop and sensory loss on the dorsum of the foot.
    (b) The tone of muscles supplied by the injured nerve will be increased.
    (c) Neurotmesis is frequently caused by compression of a nerve.
    (d) A tourniquet applied to the upper arm may result in wrist drop.
    (e) Ulnar nerve compression of the elbow causes loss of sensation over the thenar eminence.

14. *A pharyngeal pouch:*
    (a) Is a posteromedial pulsion diverticulum of the inferior constrictor muscle of the pharynx.
    (b) Usually presents with vomiting.
    (c) Is readily diagnosed by fibre-optic endoscopy.
    (d) Should be treated surgically.
    (e) Is caused by an oesophageal stricture.

15. *Non-union of a fracture:*
    (a) May be due to internal fixation.
    (b) Is more common in compound fractures.
    (c) May be associated with a pathological fracture.
    (d) Can be treated by bone grafting.
    (e) Cannot be diagnosed clinically.

16. *Following childbirth, urinary incontinence:*
    (a) Can be treated with alpha blockers such as phenoxybenzamine.
    (b) Is more common after caesarian section.
    (c) May be treated by physiotherapy.
    (d) Is most often due to urinary-tract infection.
    (e) Occurs when coughing or straining and is associated with loss of bladder neck angle.

17. *Intussusception in children:*
    (a) Has a peak incidence at about 6 months.
    (b) Is usually associated with an underlying polyp.
    (c) Presents with painless abdominal distension.
    (d) May be effectively treated by barium enema.
    (e) Commonly recurs even after effective treatment.

18. *In early breast cancer (without evidence of widespread metastases):*
    (a) Axillary node involvement can be judged by clinical examination.
    (b) Radiotherapy should be given to the axilla after surgical clearance if the nodes are involved.
    (c) Survival following wide local excision of the tumour (segmental mastectomy) is the same as that of simple mastectomy.

(d) The prognosis after removal of the breast tumour is related to the number of lymph nodes involved in the axilla.
   (e) Axillary node involvement is irrelevant in terms of management.

19. *The following pre-dispose to gallstone formation:*
   (a) Hyperparathyroidism.
   (b) Biliary infection.
   (c) Diabetes mellitus.
   (d) Crohn's disease.
   (e) Oral contraceptive pill.

20. *Cervical ribs:*
   (a) Are bilateral.
   (b) Originate from the transverse processes of the 7th cervical vertebra.
   (c) If symptomatic, most commonly cause neurological symptoms in the arm.
   (d) If symptomatic, most commonly cause venous compression.
   (e) Are frequently associated with a fibrous band.

21. *Healing of a surgical wound by first intention (primary healing):*
   (a) Involves at least 7 days of 'lag phase' before epithelialization occurs.
   (b) Is impaired by wound haematoma or infection.
   (c) Requires wound contraction.
   (d) Requires fibroblasts.
   (e) Results in a wound which is eventually stronger than the original tissue.

22. *Primary hyperparathyroidism:*
   (a) Frequently presents as a lump in the neck.
   (b) May be associated with normal serum calcium levels.
   (c) Is usually due to a single parathyroid adenoma.
   (d) May result from chronic renal failure.
   (e) Most commonly presents with osteitis fibrosa cystica.

23. *Pituitary adenomas:*
    (a) May present with bitemporal hemianopia.
    (b) Commonly become malignant.
    (c) May present with Cushing's syndrome.
    (d) Generally require frontal craniotomy to be removed.
    (e) Can cause enlargement of the pituitary fossa, apparent on plain skull X-ray.

24. *Malignant melanoma:*
    (a) Is increasing in incidence.
    (b) Is most effectively treated by radiotherapy.
    (c) Is more common in women.
    (d) Prognosis is related to vertical thickness.
    (e) Invariably arises from a pre-existing naevus.

25. *Glucocorticoid steroids:*
    (a) Are given topically to reduce the inflammatory response in cellulitis.
    (b) Cause sodium retention by the kidney.
    (c) May produce glycosuria.
    (d) May reduce intracranial pressure from cerebral oedema.
    (e) May mask the clinical signs usually associated with peritonitis.

26. *In a patient suspected of having a post-operative pulmonary embolism (PE):*
    (a) The source of embolism is most likely to be the lower limb or pelvic veins.
    (b) If the patient survives a further PE is unlikely.
    (c) A normal perfusion scan makes the diagnosis very unlikely.
    (d) Surgical removal of the embolus may occasionally be life-saving.
    (e) Heparin is only given if the source of embolus is identified as a venous thrombus.

27. *Acute small bowel obstruction:*
    (a) Is most commonly caused by carcinoma of the caecum.
    (b) Is characterized by dilated bowel seen peripherally on the plain abdominal X-ray.

(c) Presents with constipation as the first symptom.
(d) Produces a fluid thrill on abdominal examination.
(e) Requires laparotomy if not settling on conservative measures after 24–48 hours.

28. *Fractures in children:*
    (a) Which involve the epiphyseal plate must be treated conservatively to prevent interference with future bone growth.
    (b) Should not be treated by internal fixation as it impairs bone development.
    (c) Pathological fractures can occur.
    (d) A compound fracture is one which involves another major structure.
    (e) Fractures of the femoral shaft are usually treated with splintage and traction.

29. *Sigmoid volvulus:*
    (a) Is less likely in patients who take a high-fibre diet.
    (b) Usually results from trauma.
    (c) Presents with abdominal pain, intestinal obstruction and distension.
    (d) Is diagnosed by abdominal X-rays.
    (e) Usually requires emergency laparotomy.

30. *Signs suggesting the possibility of intra-abdominal malignancy include:*
    (a) Palpable umbilical lymph node.
    (b) Palpable right supraclavicular lymph node.
    (c) Shifting dullness.
    (d) Hepatomegaly.
    (e) Campbell-de-Morgan spots on the skin.

31. *Tracheostomy:*
    (a) May be indicated in a patient with facial injuries.
    (b) Involves the trachea being opened just above the second ring.
    (c) May be complicated by tracheal stenosis.
    (d) Must be performed under general anaesthesia.

(e) Requires the trachea to be closed surgically on removal of the tube.

32. *Effective management of the jaundiced patient may include:*
    (a) High protein diet.
    (b) Intravenous fluids.
    (c) Heparin.
    (d) Benzyl penicillin.
    (e) Chlorpheniramine.

33. *Fallot's tetralogy:*
    (a) Comprises pulmonary valve stenosis and a ventricular septal defect (VSD) as the primary lesions.
    (b) Is associated with Down's syndrome.
    (c) Produces finger clubbing.
    (d) Can usually be managed conservatively with drugs.
    (e) May be complicated by cerebral thrombosis.

34. *Carcinoma of the penis:*
    (a) May metastasize to the inguinal lymph nodes.
    (b) Commonly occurs in young uncircumcised men.
    (c) May be treated by local irradiation.
    (d) Is a contraindication to circumcision.
    (e) Is an adenocarcinoma arising from periurethral glands.

35. *Fracture of the humerus in an adult:*
    (a) Does not usually require open reduction.
    (b) The ulnar nerve is the commonest associated structure to be injured.
    (c) Internal fixation is generally undertaken if there is an associated fracture of the elbow joint.
    (d) The injured arm should be supported in a sling after reduction of the fracture.
    (e) Delayed union is more likely in a transverse fracture.

36. *Fractures of the radius and ulna:*
    (a) Will require internal fixation, otherwise loss of function will occur.

(b) After reduction should be immobilized in a plaster from the axilla to the metacarpal heads.
(c) Greenstick fractures in children require no treatment.
(d) Volkmann's ischaemia may occur in the absence of major arterial injury.
(e) Compound fractures should be plated.

37. *Hodgkin's disease:*
    (a) Usually presents with inguinal lymphadenopathy and splenomegaly.
    (b) Is characterized by enlarged lymph nodes that are stony hard on palpation.
    (c) Is characterized histologically by the appearance of Reed–Sternberg cells.
    (d) If classified as lymphocyte-predominant carries the best prognosis.
    (e) Is treated by radical surgical excision.

38. *Following routine tonsillectomy:*
    (a) Bleeding at 7–10 days is common and requires no active treatment.
    (b) Earache is relatively common.
    (c) Patients will be more prone to pneumococcal chest infections.
    (d) Primary haemorrhage can be treated with antibiotics.
    (e) Antibiotic prophylaxis should be maintained for 7 days.

39. *Colorectal cancer:*
    (a) Has a peak incidence in 50-year-olds.
    (b) Of the right colon usually presents with rectal bleeding.
    (c) Usually presents with acute obstruction when left-sided.
    (d) Spreads locally in a mainly longitudinal fashion, up and down the bowel lumen.
    (e) Carries a prognosis that is related to the extent of local and lymph node spread.

40. *A patient undergoing amputation of the leg for advanced ischaemia:*
    (a) Will achieve better mobility with a below-knee amputation.
    (b) Will be more likely to achieve primary healing with a below-knee amputation.
    (c) May use an inflatable prosthetic limb to achieve early mobility.
    (d) May develop phantom limb pain that improves if re-amputation is performed at a higher level.
    (e) Should be given antibiotics prophylactically.

41. *In a motorcyclist, thrown from his machine and landing on his left shoulder and head:*
    (a) A completely paralysed left arm suggests a spinal cord injury.
    (b) If the arm is held internally rotated and pronated a C5 and C6 root injury of the brachial plexus is likely.
    (c) If complete avulsion of the brachial plexus has occurred urgent surgical repair should be undertaken.
    (d) A left-sided Horner's syndrome and paralysed arm has a bad prognosis for recovery of arm function.
    (e) The transverse processes of the cervical vertebrae may be fractured.

42. *In a patient with a suspected phaeochromocytoma:*
    (a) Hypotension can occur.
    (b) The diagnosis can be confirmed using intravenous beta blockers.
    (c) Urinary vanillymandelic acid (VMA) is increased.
    (d) Computerized tomography (CT) scan will often locate the tumour.
    (e) The tumours are benign.

43. *Venous ulcers:*
    (a) May occur after a deep vein thrombosis (DVT).
    (b) Are uncommon in men.
    (c) Must be treated medically prior to surgical intervention.
    (d) Can be treated with hydrocolloid dressings.
    (e) Should initially be excised and skin grafted.

44. *Failure to pass motion in a new-born baby:*
    (a) Is most likely due to constipation.
    (b) Plain X-rays may help determine the cause.
    (c) A thin membrane may cover the anus.
    (d) Due to a congenital rectal abnormality increases the chance of urinary-tract problems.
    (e) May be associated with a fistula.

45. *Venous ulcers of the lower limb:*
    (a) Are commonly seen above the medial malleolus at the ankle.
    (b) If infected should be treated with topical antibiotics.
    (c) Are invariably secondary to occluded deep veins following deep venous thrombosis (DVT).
    (d) Once clean, should be treated by compression bandages and elevation.
    (e) Are prevented from recurring by long-term anticoagulant therapy.

46. *An inguinal hernia:*
    (a) In childhood, should be treated expectantly as many resolve.
    (b) Controlled by pressure over the deep inguinal ring is likely to be indirect.
    (c) May include the testicle in the sac.
    (d) Does not occur in women as they have no inguinal canal.
    (e) Is rarely bilateral.

47. *Concerning a palpable lump in the parotid region:*
    (a) Excision biopsy of the lump should be performed to exclude malignancy.
    (b) If the lump is a pleomorphic adenoma, superficial parotidectomy should be undertaken.
    (c) If the lump is an enlarged lymph node it can be safely left.
    (d) Fine-needle aspiration cytology (FNAC) may give a pre-operative diagnosis.
    (e) Ipsilateral facial nerve palsy makes it more likely that the lump is malignant.

48. *In a young man with a fractured shaft of femur:*
    (a) Palpable pedal pulses recorded on admission excludes significant arterial injury.
    (b) Absent pulses are usually due to arterial spasm.
    (c) If the patient is hypotensive with an expanding haematoma in the thigh, angiography should be arranged.
    (d) If significant arterial and venous injuries are found temporary shunts may be used while fracture fixation is performed.
    (e) Injured veins are usually ligated.

49. *Squamous cell carcinoma of the skin:*
    (a) Presents as an irregular ulcer with an indurated base and raised everted edges.
    (b) Readily metastasizes to regional lymph nodes.
    (c) Is characterized by early blood-borne spread to the liver and lungs.
    (d) May develop in a chronic venous leg ulcer.
    (e) Is not found in areas of the body not regularly exposed to sunlight.

50. *Anal fissure:*
    (a) Produces severe pain during and immediately after defaecation.
    (b) Is usually associated with Crohns' disease.
    (c) Usually occurs in the midline posteriorly.
    (d) Is effectively treated by sclerotherapy.
    (e) May be treated by division of the lower fibres of the internal sphincter muscle.

Paper 5

1. *A 70-year-old man presenting with general malaise, weight loss and irregular hepatomegaly:*
   (a) Is likely to have an advanced malignancy.
   (b) Should probably have a liver biopsy.
   (c) Should have a progressive series of radiological and endoscopic investigations to establish the site of the primary tumour.
   (d) Needs a prolonged stay in a surgical ward to restore normal body physiology and nutrition.
   (e) May benefit from radiotherapy.

2. *In a teenager presenting with an acutely painful, swollen testicle:*
   (a) Epididymo-orchitis is the most likely diagnosis.
   (b) Clinical examination can usually exclude the diagnosis of torsion.
   (c) Horizontal lie of the testicles increases the risk of torsion.
   (d) Manual detorsion may be effective treatment.
   (e) Emergency surgical exploration is invariably indicated.

3. *Secondary bone tumours:*
   (a) Osteolytic lesions are the most frequent.
   (b) Breast and prostate carcinomas are the commonest primaries to metastasize to bone.
   (c) Internal fixation is contraindicated.
   (d) Local radiotherapy can reduce pain.
   (e) The primary tumour must be identified.

4. *A breast lump presenting in a 22-year-old woman:*
   (a) Should be investigated further by mammography.
   (b) Is probably a cyst and can safely be ignored.
   (c) Fine-needle aspiration cytology (FNAC) may determine the nature of the lump.

(d) Is most likely to be a fibroadenoma.
(e) Is more likely if the woman is on the oral contraceptive pill.

5. *Accepted indications for laparoscopic cholecystectomy include:*
   (a) Asymptomatic gallstones in a 40-year-old woman.
   (b) Jaundice associated with severe acute pancreatitis that is failing to resolve.
   (c) Fatty food intolerance.
   (d) Biliary colic.
   (e) Acute cholecystitis.

6. *Meningiomas:*
   (a) May present with epilepsy.
   (b) Commonly metastasize to the skull.
   (c) May cause papilloedema.
   (d) Should be treated by surgical removal in most cases.
   (e) May be apparent on skull X-ray.

7. *Oedema of one leg:*
   (a) May be caused by pelvic malignancy.
   (b) Is most commonly due to heart failure.
   (c) Due to lymphatic hypoplasia may not present until adulthood.
   (d) Is rarely due to venous obstruction.
   (e) Usually requires surgical treatment.

8. *Successful renal transplantation:*
   (a) Is more likely when the donor kidney is taken from a living relative than from a cadaver.
   (b) Is unlikely in the presence of ABO incompatibility.
   (c) Is only possible with at least three HLA haplotypes identical between donor and recipient.
   (d) Risks subsequent malignancy.
   (e) Is achieved in 30% of recipients 5 years after transplant surgery.

9. *In a patient who has had a transient weakness of the left arm:*
    (a) Carotid angiography should be arranged.
    (b) Anticoagulation with heparin is commenced.
    (c) If a mild (10%) atheromatous stenosis of the right internal carotid artery is found oral aspirin is indicated.
    (d) Carotid duplex scanning of the carotids should be obtained.
    (e) Carotid artery disease is the most likely cause of this event.

10. *The treatment of haemorrhoids:*
    (a) By simple outpatient methods is associated with a high recurrence rate, and in a young person formal haemorrhoidectomy is indicated in most cases.
    (b) By injection sclerotherapy with phenol is suitable for first-degree piles.
    (c) By rubber-band ligation is useful for chronic, prolapsed piles that have become covered with skin.
    (d) By anal dilatation is indicated in elderly patients.
    (e) By haemorrhoidectomy may be complicated by anal stenoses.

11. *Chronic osteomyelitis:*
    (a) May complicate a compound fracture of the tibia.
    (b) An abscess cavity may be seen on X-ray.
    (c) Often presents as a pathological fracture.
    (d) Is associated with bone necrosis.
    (e) May recur after many years.

12. *A child with posterior urethral valves:*
    (a) May have been diagnosed prior to birth.
    (b) Presents with a jet-like stream on micturition.
    (c) May be treated by endoscopic resection of the valves.
    (d) May present with a urinary-tract infection.
    (e) Will be impossible to catheterize per-urethrally due to the valves.

13. *Haemorrhoids:*
    (a) Represent varicosities of the superior rectal veins.
    (b) Are common in pregnancy.
    (c) May be avoided by taking a high-fibre diet.
    (d) Usually present with pain on defaecation.
    (e) Can be felt on *per rectum* examination at '3, 7 and 11 o'clock'.

14. *Patients with intermittent claudication:*
    (a) Should be encouraged to stop smoking.
    (b) Are very likely to progress to limb-threatening ischaemia.
    (c) May be diagnosed by measuring systolic ankle blood pressure before and after exercise.
    (d) Usually improve their walking ability with vasoactive drugs.
    (e) If overweight, weight loss will improve their walking.

15. *In a patient in atrial fibrillation presenting with shock and severe abdominal pain:*
    (a) Mesenteric embolus is unlikely if abdominal signs of peritonitis are absent.
    (b) A high white-cell count and metabolic acidosis strongly suggest a severely ischaemic bowel.
    (c) Laparotomy is unnecessary if the serum amylase is raised.
    (d) Laparotomy should be delayed until the acid–base balance and renal function have been corrected.
    (e) Complete recovery is usual after mesenteric embolectomy.

16. *In rheumatoid arthritis (RA):*
    (a) The primary pathology is destruction of the articular cartilage.
    (b) There may be a rapid onset associated with widespread lymphadenopathy.
    (c) Subcutaneous nodules are sometimes found.
    (d) Rheumatoid factor is non-specific.
    (e) Steroids are often indicated.

17. *In a 60-year-old man presenting acutely with profuse, bright red per rectum bleeding:*
    (a) Colonic carcinoma is the most likely diagnosis.
    (b) Procto-sigmoidoscopy should be performed after initial resuscitation.
    (c) Emergency barium enema is indicated if sigmoidoscopy is negative.
    (d) Mesenteric angiography should be performed after the bleeding has stopped.
    (e) If due to angiodysplasia, bleeding is most likely to originate from the right colon.

18. *Endoscopic retrograde cholangio-pancreatography (ERCP):*
    (a) May be indicated before laparoscopic cholecystectomy in patients with abnormal liver function tests.
    (b) Is the first-line investigation in patients with jaundice.
    (c) Is contraindicated in jaundiced patients with acute pancreatitis.
    (d) Should be utilized cautiously as it carries a mortality of over 10%.
    (e) Is useful in the diagnosis and treatment of biliary malignancy.

19. *In a patient undergoing angiography of an ischaemic lower limb:*
    (a) Absence of the femoral pulse makes angiography impossible.
    (b) A Seldinger catheter placement technique via the ipsilateral femoral artery is the method of choice.
    (c) Intravenous digital subtraction angiography (IV-DSA) is of no value.
    (d) Antibiotic prophylaxis is used if the patient has gangrene.
    (e) Embolization of atheroma is a recognized complication.

20. *Total parenteral nutrition (TPN):*
    (a) Is indicated before most major abdominal surgery to improve wound healing and recovery.

(b) May be given via a fine-bore nasogastric tube.
(c) Is invaluable in severely ill patients with multi-organ failure and post-operative catabolism.
(d) Usually requires a central venous cannula.
(e) Should be of high-calorie, low-protein, low-fat composition.

21. *A cystic hygroma:*
    (a) Is frequently mistaken for a thyroglossal cyst.
    (b) Does not usually present until adolescence.
    (c) Is malignant.
    (d) Should be treated by radiotherapy.
    (e) Is seen most frequently in the base of the posterior triangle of the neck.

22. *Necrotizing enterocolitis (NEC) in a neonate:*
    (a) Is more common in premature babies.
    (b) May present with bloody stools.
    (c) Rarely causes bowel perforation.
    (d) Bowel resection may be required.
    (e) Is due to infection with *Escherichia coli*.

23. *Pruritis ani in adults:*
    (a) May be a manifestation of proctitis.
    (b) Is usually due to threadworm infection.
    (c) May respond to advice on anal hygiene and cleansing.
    (d) Is effectively treated by topical application of strong steroid cream (e.g. Betnovate).
    (e) May be helped by wearing loose cotton underwear.

24. *Carcinoma of the pancreas:*
    (a) Is associated with chronic pancreatitis.
    (b) Often presents with pain.
    (c) Carries a better prognosis than cancer of the ampulla of Vater.
    (d) Has a 5-year survival rate of 40%.
    (e) Is associated with smoking.

25. *In a patient suffering from ureteric colic:*
    (a) Severe pain is usually associated with pyrexia.

(b) Calculi are usually seen on a plain X-ray.
   (c) Opiates are the only effective analgesics.
   (d) A high fluid load should be administered to 'flush out' the stone.
   (e) An urgent intravenous urogram (IVU) is usually diagnostic.

26. *Ankylosing spondylitis (AS):*
    (a) Commonly affects the cervical spine in the early stages.
    (b) Fibrosis and ossification of the intervertebral discs can occur.
    (c) X-ray appearances of erosion of the sacroiliac joints appear early in the disease.
    (d) There is a strong association with HLA-B27 antigen.
    (e) Most often presents in elderly men.

27. *A fistula-in-ano (anal fistula):*
    (a) Usually originates from a perianal abscess.
    (b) Presents with severe pain after defaecation.
    (c) With the external opening anteriorly, communicates with the anal canal directly (the internal opening is seen at the same radius).
    (d) May be associated with Crohn's disease.
    (e) Usually heals spontaneously with antibiotic treatment.

28. *Salivary gland calculi:*
    (a) Most commonly cause symptoms in the submandibular gland.
    (b) May cause pain on eating.
    (c) Require the affected gland to be removed.
    (d) Are associated with increased risk of malignancy.
    (e) May occur secondarily to abnormal calcium metabolism.

29. *Following a femoropopliteal artery (below-knee) bypass:*
    (a) Occlusion of the bypass might be expected to occur in 10–20% of patients in the first year.
    (b) If the patient's saphenous vein is used, a stenosis may develop in up to 30% of grafts.
    (c) Aspirin therapy is of no value.

(d) The results using prosthetic bypass material are the same as if the long saphenous vein is used.
(e) Graft failure after 4 years is most likely due to progression of atheroma in the patient's native arteries.

30. *Irritable bowel syndrome (IBS):*
    (a) Can be confidently diagnosed on history alone.
    (b) Usually presents with bloody diarrhoea.
    (c) Is often alleviated by a low residue diet.
    (d) Results from an absence of Meissner's plexuses in the abnormal bowel.
    (e) May respond to life-style changes.

31. *Bladder tumours:*
    (a) T1 transitional cell carcinomas are treated by resection of the tumour alone.
    (b) Total cystectomy may be required for advanced or frequently recurrent tumours.
    (c) Smoking is an associated risk factor.
    (d) Adenocarcinomas are the most common type.
    (e) Schistosomiasis may cause bladder tumours.

32. *In a 5-year-old boy with suspected acute osteomyelitis:*
    (a) The site of the bone infection is usually the metaphysis.
    (b) There will generally be signs of penetrating injury over the bone involved.
    (c) *Staphylococci* are the commonest organisms involved.
    (d) X-rays of the area are diagnostic.
    (e) Surgical drainage may be required.

33. *Symptoms and signs characteristic of peritonitis include:*
    (a) Reflex bradycardia.
    (b) Vomiting.
    (c) Pyrexia.
    (d) Abdominal rigidity.
    (e) Increased bowel sounds.

34. *In a 70-year-old man presenting with haematemesis:*
    (a) Hospital admission is required.

(b) Upper gastrointestinal endoscopy should be carried out as soon as possible after initial resuscitation.
(c) The source of bleeding may be identified and bleeding arrested via the endoscope.
(d) If bleeding continues, the threshold for surgical intervention is higher than for a younger patient, due to the high risk of surgery.
(e) The cause is likely to be oesophageal varices.

35. *Following a successful aortic aneurysm repair:*
    (a) Patients require antibiotic prophylaxis for dental extractions.
    (b) Anticoagulation with warfarin will be continued for life.
    (c) Further aneurysms develop in over 50% of patients.
    (d) Haematemesis may be due to an aortoduodenal fistula.
    (e) The graft life-expectancy is 5–10 years.

36. *In an elderly woman presenting with a strangulated femoral hernia:*
    (a) Intestinal obstruction is invariably present.
    (b) The hernia is tender.
    (c) The white-cell count is usually raised.
    (d) Urgent surgery is indicated after resuscitation.
    (e) Repair under local anaesthetic may be possible.

37. *In a patient who has suffered a blow to the head, but not lost consciousness:*
    (a) Admission to hospital will not be required.
    (b) A rising pulse rate and hypotension are signs of increasing intracranial pressure.
    (c) Computerized tomography (CT) scanning may reveal unsuspected haematomas.
    (d) A depressed skull fracture must be elevated.
    (e) Rhinorrhoea is an indication for antibiotics.

38. *Patients with transitional cell bladder tumours:*
    (a) May present with anaemia.
    (b) Usually present with haematuria.

(c) Have a low recurrence rate after primary treatment.
(d) May respond to chemotherapy.
(e) The disease can be staged using ultrasound.

39. *Patients with Menière's disease:*
    (a) Generally have a history of chronic ear disease.
    (b) Complain of tinitis.
    (c) Suffer a steady, gradual decline in hearing ability.
    (d) May have no response to caloric labyrinthine function testing.
    (e) Have neurosensory hearing impairment.

40. *In a patient with a popliteal artery aneurysm (PAA):*
    (a) The surgical treatment is to bypass the PAA and ligate the popliteal artery above and below (exclusion bypass).
    (b) The risk of rupture is high.
    (c) Presentation may be with an acutely ischaemic leg.
    (d) Thrombolysis with streptokinase may be used in the treatment.
    (e) Conservative treatment may be an option.

41. *Bunions:*
    (a) Are due to a prominent first metatarsal head.
    (b) May be seen in adolescence.
    (c) Are associated with rheumatoid arthritis.
    (d) Excision arthroplasty is often undertaken.
    (e) Are rarely painful.

42. *In a 75-year-old man with a 7 cm diameter abdominal aortic aneurysm:*
    (a) Repair should be undertaken only if the aneurysm is symptomatic.
    (b) Repair involves resection of the aneurysm sac.
    (c) The prognosis for the patient after successful surgery returns to that of a 'normal' 75-year-old.
    (d) The expected mortality rate of elective surgery will be in excess of 15%.
    (e) Renal artery involvement is not a contraindication to surgery.

43. *Rupture of the Achilles tendon:*
    (a) Tends to occur in young people during periods of prolonged sporting activity.
    (b) Should not be treated surgically.
    (c) The diagnosis can be confirmed by squeezing the calf of the prone patient.
    (d) The foot should be held in plantar flexion while healing occurs.
    (e) The patient may complain that they were hit from behind at the time of injury.

44. *Diverticular disease of the colon:*
    (a) Results from high segmental pressures of the colon.
    (b) Usually remains asymptomatic.
    (c) May present with symptoms and signs similar to those of acute appendicitis.
    (d) When perforated, causing faecal peritonitis, requires laparotomy and suture of the perforated diverticulum.
    (e) Complicated by acute diverticulitis, often settles with conservative measures.

45. *In a 16-year-old girl complaining of pain around the knee:*
    (a) Dislocation of the patella may occur spontaneously without a precipitating injury.
    (b) Degenerative changes in the articular cartilage of the patella (chondromalacia) may cause pain.
    (c) Osgood–Schlatter's disease rarely occurs in this age group.
    (d) If lateral pressure on the patella during knee flexion causes resistance or discomfort the most likely cause of the pain is a meniscal injury.
    (e) If a stellate fracture of the patella is found this is an indication for patellectomy.

46. *Epididymal cysts:*
    (a) Are often multiple.
    (b) May cause subfertility and should be removed.
    (c) Can be effectively treated with sclerosant.
    (d) Can be palpated in front of the testicle.
    (e) May be safely left.

47. *Circumcision in children:*
    (a) Is indicated for the treatment of phimosis.
    (b) Should be performed after an episode of balanitis in an infant.
    (c) Should be performed if the foreskin is still non-retractile at the age of 3 years.
    (d) May reduce the risk of subsequent carcinoma of the penis.
    (e) Is readily performed under local anaesthetic.

48. *Acute pancreatitis is frequently complicated by:*
    (a) Non-cardiogenic pulmonary oedema.
    (b) Diabetes mellitus.
    (c) Hypercalcaemia.
    (d) A collection of fluid in the lesser sac.
    (e) Bacterial septicaemia.

49. *Causes of chronic foul-smelling aural discharge in an adult include:*
    (a) A foreign body.
    (b) Acute otitis media.
    (c) Perforation of the ear drum.
    (d) External otitis.
    (e) Cholesteatoma.

50. *A false aneurysm in the femoral artery:*
    (a) May follow an angiogram.
    (b) Is most often due to atherosclerosis.
    (c) Will thrombose spontaneously in most cases.
    (d) May be mistaken for a haematoma.
    (e) Is treated by ligation of the artery.

Answers to Paper 1

1. (a) F.
   (b) F.
   (c) T.
   (d) F.
   (e) T.

   Most abdominal aortic aneurysms are asymptomatic and abdominal examination is unreliable, hence the rationale of screening programmes using ultrasound scanning. Aneurysms are more common in men (male/female 4:1), although the relative incidence in women is increasing. First-degree relatives of patients with aneurysms are 3–8 times more likely to have an aneurysm themselves and patients with peripheral vascular disease are approximately 4 times more likely to have an aneurysm than the general population.

2. (a) F.
   (b) T.
   (c) F.
   (d) F.
   (e) T.

   Adenocarcinoma of the oesophagus is the commonest tumour found in the lower third of the oesophagus and may arise within the area of 'Barrett's' columnar-lined oesophagus. It is not radiosensitive and subtotal oesophagectomy offers the only chance of 'cure' or extended palliation. Prognosis is even worse than that for squamous cell carcinoma and remains at under 10% at 5 years. Squamous tumours are commoner in the upper two-thirds of the oesophagus, respond more readily to radiotherapy and may rarely complicate achalasia.

Oesophageal carcinoma cannot be confidently excluded by barium swallow, endoscopy and biopsy being essential in the investigation of dysphagia.

3. (a) F.
   (b) T.
   (c) F.
   (d) F.
   (e) F.

CABG is indicated in patients with severe angina not relieved by medical treatment. It is a safe procedure with a mortality of around 2% and usually provides excellent symptomatic relief. It may also prolong life in some patients with severe disease and poor left ventricular function. The IMA and LSV are the conduits of choice and prosthetic grafts are not used as the vessel diameters are too small. Angioplasty may be effective in the treatment of short stenoses but restenosis rates are high and the disease is often too advanced for it to be possible.

4. (a) T.
   (b) F.
   (c) T.
   (d) F.
   (e) T.

Several severity scores have been described based mainly on laboratory criteria. The presence of more than three criteria indicates a severe attack. These include: age >55 years, WCC >16 × 10^9/l, serum albumin <32 g/l, serum calcium <2.0 mmol/l, aspartate aminotransferase >100 IU/l, lactate dehydrogenase >600 IU/l, blood glucose >10.0 mmol/l, blood urea >16 mmol/l and P_aO_2 < 7.5 kPa. A very high serum amylase is diagnostic but carries no prognostic significance. Ultrasound may detect gallstones or fluid collections, but will not otherwise predict severity.

5. (a) T.
   (b) F.

(c) F.
(d) F.
(e) T.
Oesophagitis usually results from the reflux of acidic stomach contents into the oesophagus. This is associated with decreased lower oesophageal sphincter (LOS) tone and may or may not accompany hiatus hernia. Reflux commonly presents with heartburn, but chronic inflammation may result in stricture formation and dysphagia. Bile reflux is an uncommon cause of oesophagitis and usually follows gastric surgery. Treatment of reflux symptoms includes simple life-style advice, antacids, alginates, drugs which increase LOS tone (metoclopramide or cisapride) and H_2-receptor antagonists. Acute, severe oesophagitis, however, is most effectively managed by omeprazole. Antireflux surgery such as fundoplication is reserved for failed medical management or complications.

6. (a) F.
   (b) F.
   (c) F.
   (d) T.
   (e) T.
Episodes of acute disc protrusion are often preceded by minor episodes of backache. The acute episode often subsides. The commonest disc to be effected is L5/S1, followed by L4/5. Males are affected 4 times more commonly than females. Diagnosis is usually based on history and examination, but computerized tomography (CT) scan and, in particular, MRI give clear views of the affected disc and avoid myelography with its potential complications. Protrusion of the L4/5 disc can cause compression of the 5th lumbar nerve root with weakness of big toe and knee extension with brisk knee jerks due to the weak antagonists. Anterior disc protrusion may compress the cauda equina with urinary retention and sensory loss over the sacrum.

7. (a) F.
   (b) F.
   (c) T.
   (d) T.
   (e) F.
   Ureteric stones almost always cause haematuria, although this may be microscopic and only be apparent on testing. They occur twice as often in males as in females. Infection in the renal tract above the stone is an indication for removal of the stone. So are failure of the stone to progress, persistent pain and worsening ipsilateral renal function. 90% of stones are apparent on plain X-ray, but an intravenous urogram is necessary to confirm the diagnosis. Two per cent of renal stones are due to cystinuria. Cystine stone formation can be reduced by penicillamine, which forms a soluble complex with cystine, but this will not dissolve formed stones.

8. (a) F.
   (b) F.
   (c) T.
   (d) F.
   (e) T.
   Mammographic screening began in the UK after the recommendations of the Forrest report in 1987, with the intention of improving the early diagnosis of breast cancer. All women aged 50–65 years are invited to undergo single oblique view mammography of each breast every 3 years. The incidence of breast carcinoma is less in pre-menopausal women, and cancers in this group are less likely to be visible on mammography. Women with suspicious mammograms (about 6% of the total) are recalled for further X-rays, clinical examination and/or fine needle aspiration cytology for palpable lumps. Less than 1% of women screened undergo surgical biopsy (directed by wires inserted under X-ray control for impalpable lesions), and two cancers are discovered for every benign lesion excised.

ANSWERS TO PAPER ONE

9. (a) T.
   (b) F.
   (c) T.
   (d) F.
   (e) T.
   Compression of the median nerve at the wrist usually causes pain in the middle and index fingers, worse at night, and relieved by moving or shaking the hand. There is not usually any obvious cause for the condition, but it can occur in pregnancy, hypothyroidism, tenosynovitis and rheumatoid arthritis. Weakness of thumb abduction and thenar wasting are not usually the presenting symptom but may be present. The clinical diagnosis is not always clear-cut and should be confirmed prior to surgical decompression. Other methods of treatment include temporary splintage and steroid injections into the canal.

10. (a) T.
    (b) F.
    (c) T.
    (d) T.
    (e) F.
    Fractured NOF is a very common cause of admission to hospital, especially in elderly females as the fracture occurs to weak osteoporotic bone. The fracture is obviously painful but the leg is usually shortened and externally rotated due to the unopposed action of the psoas muscle. The complications of prolonged bed-rest in the elderly mean that early internal fixation of the fracture is the treatment of choice in the majority of cases, but mortality remains very high as the presence of a fractured NOF may be an indication of the generally poor physical condition of the patient.

11. (a) F.
    (b) F.
    (c) T.
    (d) F.
    (e) T.

Duodenal ulceration is commonly associated with a basal, nocturnal and stimulated increase in gastric acidity, and hence reduction with H_2-receptor antagonists usually leads to healing. Subsequent recurrence, however, is not uncommon and such ulcers may be associated with *Helicobacter* which should then be treated with 'triple therapy' of antibiotics and De-nol. The incidence of peptic ulceration has been declining since before the introduction of cimetidine. Malignancy should always be excluded in stomach ulcers, but duodenal ulcers are invariably benign.

12. (a) F.
    (b) T.
    (c) F.
    (d) F.
    (e) T.

In 80% of claudicants symptoms remain stable or improve, although 50% will die over the following 10 years from coronary or cerebrovascular disease. Angiography will identify arterial stenoses and occlusions, but it is invasive and does not confirm that the pain on walking is due to arterial insufficiency. This should be done by measurement of resting and post-exercise ankle systolic blood pressures measurement. Supervised exercise is currently the only non-surgical treatment of proven benefit, sympathectomy has no proven benefit. Transluminal angioplasty is widely used, but whether it is better than exercise alone remains controversial.

13. (a) F.
    (b) F.
    (c) F.
    (d) T.
    (e) F.

Children and young adults usually present with indirect herniae due to a congenital sac; direct herniation is more likely in older patients with weakened posterior inguinal walls. There are very few contraindications to elective hernia repair as operation under local anaesthetic is possible; trusses rarely control the hernia and the risk of incarceration remains. Many patients with inguinal hernias are suitable for day-case surgery and early mobilization is encouraged. Monofilament, non-absorbable sutures are required to effect permanent repair of the posterior inguinal wall, and infection rates are low.

14. (a) F.
    (b) T.
    (c) F.
    (d) F.
    (e) F.
    NTNG is the most common cause of a generalized thyroid swelling. It is usually seen in middle-aged women. The aetiology is unclear but the thyroid consists of areas of degeneration, hyperplasia, cystic change and fibrosis. It is *not* the endemic goitre of iodine deficiency (now unknown in the UK since the iodization of salt) or the self-limiting 'physiological' goitre of menarche or pregnancy. 'Non-toxic', by definition, implies that the patient is euthyroid. Indications for surgery (subtotal thyroidectomy) are for complications, including compression of the trachea, and patient discomfort or anxiety over the appearance. NTNG is not a pre-malignant condition, but may be surgically removed if malignancy cannot be excluded.

15. (a) F.
    (b) F.
    (c) T.
    (d) F.
    (e) F.
    Traditional regimens of 'PRN' intramuscular opiates provide poor analgesia, certainly when short-acting drugs are given many hours apart. Intravenous infusions of opiates, especially when combined with 'on-demand' bolus doses (patient-controlled analgesia), are more effective. Oral analgesics cannot be given in the early post-operative period after major abdominal surgery. Regional analgesia such as an epidural infusion or non-steroidal anti-inflammatory drugs (NSAIDs), including diclofenac

suppositories, both reduce opiate requirements. It is desirable that the patient awakes from the anaesthetic pain-free, and local infiltration of the wound with bupivacaine is valuable.

16. (a) F.
    (b) T.
    (c) T.
    (d) F.
    (e) F.

Exposure to ultraviolet light is the major risk factor for the development of malignant melanoma, but dark-skinned races are relatively immune (negros may develop melanomas on the lesser-pigmented soles of the feet, however). Thus, those at highest risk are fair-skinned people living in hot climates (e.g. Australia) and a history of frequent sunburn increases the risk further. Melanomas may occur in pre-existing naevi and individuals with many moles are therefore at risk. Melanomas are almost unknown before puberty and most commonly present in the 3rd to 5th decades. Smoking is not a recognized risk factor.

17. (a) T.
    (b) F.
    (c) F.
    (d) T.
    (e) T.

Hydrocephalus may be due to obstruction of flow of CSF or overproduction/failure to reabsorb the fluid. In children congenital abnormalities of the aqueduct, scarring following infection or intracranial bleeding and tumours are the commonest causes. In older patients tumours tend to be more common, although in some adults with dilated ventricles the CSF pressure is found to be normal. It may be possible to bypass the blockage, but commonly a 'shunt' is inserted to drain CSF from the lateral ventricle via a unidirectional valve into either the central venous system or the peritoneal cavity. Long-standing raised intracranial pressure may cause thinning of the skull which may be seen on X-ray (beaten silver).

18. (a) F.
    (b) T.
    (c) F.
    (d) T.
    (e) F.

Acute lower abdominal pain in a young woman may be due to appendicitis, but non-specific abdominal pain or gynaecological pathology are more likely. Laparoscopy may avoid laparotomy when there is clinical doubt and might also permit definitive treatment. X-rays are superfluous unless intestinal obstruction or visceral perforation is suspected. Rovsing's sign (pressure applied to the left iliac fossa producing pain in the right iliac fossa) does not reliably differentiate between appendicitis and gynaecological causes of peritonism. It is a myth that analgesia will mask signs of peritonitis. It is totally unacceptable to withhold analgesia from patients suffering severe pain, and effective analgesia makes examination and diagnosis easier.

19. (a) F.
    (b) F.
    (c) T.
    (d) F.
    (e) T.

Although comprising 1% of malignancies in men, cancer of the testicle is the commonest cancer in young men and 50% of cases are seminomas. There has been a 300% increase in the incidence of testicular tumours. The commonest presentation is of a testicular mass, but some men present with secondaries and an impalpable testicular tumour. Ultrasound and tumour markers (e.g. alpha-fetoprotein) usually determine the diagnosis. Metastatic potential is low and less than 25% will have extratesticular spread at the time of presentation. Para-aortic lymph nodes are most commonly involved and the inguinal nodes only become involved if the scrotum is breached, e.g. orchidectomy via the scrotum rather than via the inguinal canal. Prophylactic radiotherapy is usually given to the para-aortic region.

20. (a) T.
    (b) F.
    (c) T.
    (d) F.
    (e) T.

Presenting symptoms include discomfort in the throat, pain in the ear due to invasion of the auricular branch of the vagus nerve, and halitosis. However, the tumour may invade the larynx causing hoarseness and 50% of the tumours have spread to lymph nodes at the time of presentation. Surgical treatment usually involves pharyngolaryngectomy and radical neck dissection if lymph nodes are involved. Reconstruction of the oesophagus is undertaken either using the stomach 'pull-up' technique, a free jejunal interposition bypass, or a pectoralis flap. The tumours are squamous cell carcinomas and usually respond to radiotherapy which may be given alone for palliation or in combination with surgery. The recurrence rate for both forms of treatment tends to be high. Associated risk factors for pharyngeal carcinoma include previous radiotherapy of the neck, smoking and alcohol and, very rarely, long-standing pharyngeal pouches.

21. (a) F.
    (b) T.
    (c) T.
    (d) F.
    (e) F.

The only evidence so far established for carotid endarterectomy is for severe stenoses of the ICA (over 70%) which are symptomatic. The lesion may cause transient ischaemic attacks, amaurosis fugax (temporary loss of vision or visual disturbance due to microemboli), or permanent stroke, most likely to affect the left hemisphere

ANSWERS TO PAPER ONE

resulting in right-sided symptoms. Up to 30% of carotid artery lesions have no audible bruit and, vice versa, some bruits are not associated with arterial disease. The majority of lesions will be atheromatous.

22. (a) T.
    (b) F.
    (c) F.
    (d) T.
    (e) F.

Wound infection after abdominal surgery usually results from contamination by the patient's own bacteria and the incidence is thus higher after contaminated surgery (when the bowel is opened, for example). To achieve most effective prophylaxis, antibiotics should be given intravenously at the time of surgery. Long courses of post-operative antibiotics add nothing and encourage resistance; the role of locally applied antiseptics is unproven. When infection is established, pus should be drained, by removal of sutures and local probing at least.

23. (a) F.
    (b) F.
    (c) F.
    (d) T.
    (e) F.

Claudication is one of the earliest symptoms of lower limb peripheral vascular disease and ulcers are uncommon at this stage. An exception is a trivial injury to the foot which fails to heal and may present as an ulcer. If the arterial disease progresses perfusion of the tissues becomes reduced, especially distally, and small 'punched-out' ulcers develop on the toes and foot. Elevation of the foot further reduces the perfusion, increases the pain, and if continued will make the ulcer worse. Ischaemic ulcers mistaken for venous ulcers and treated with elevation and compression dressings will rapidly deteriorate. Unless the blood supply to the limb is improved, for example by bypass surgery or angioplasty, local surgical treatment is rarely successful. Surgical removal of the dead tissue, debridement, is often undertaken in combination with a revascularization procedure.

24. (a) T.
    (b) T.
    (c) F.
    (d) F.
    (e) F.

Solitary nodules may be truly solitary or part of occult diffuse thyroid pathology. The risk of neoplasm is much higher than for diffuse goitres and malignancies are invariably 'cold' on technetium scanning. Ultrasound may usefully identify a cyst but FNA would also, and if the lesion was found to be solid could also help plan management if a carcinoma was diagnosed. Benign lesions require only subtotal lobectomy.

25. (a) T.
    (b) F.
    (c) F.
    (d) T.
    (e) F.

Rupture of an intracranial aneurysm is the most frequent identifiable cause of SAH. Other causes include arteriovenous malformations, atherosclerosis, trauma and tumours. Approximately 20% of patients will die from the initial event, but there is a high risk of further bleeding in up to 40% during the first few weeks.

Symptoms may vary, but if bleeding is extensive rapid loss of consciousness occurs. Other symptoms include headache, vomiting, neck stiffness and photophobia.

It is important to identify treatable causes of the SAH before further bleeding occurs with angiography. The general state of the patient including level of consciousness and blood pressure must be satisfactory before undertaking the investigation and any subsequent intervention. Surgical treatment involves direct clipping of the aneurysm neck. Occasionally evacuation of intracranial haematoma may improve the situation.

26. (a) T.
    (b) F.
    (c) F.
    (d) T.
    (e) F.
    Squamous cell carcinoma of the lung accounts for more deaths in the UK than any other cancer. The best chance of cure is surgical excision by lobectomy or pneumonectomy but 75% of patients are inoperable – either they are unfit, distant metastases are present, or the tumour has spread extensively to render surgical excision impossible, e.g. to mediastinal nodes or chest wall. Radiotherapy provides the best alternative – either 'curative' or palliative for symptoms of pain, haemoptysis or superior vena caval obstruction. Chemotherapy has proved disappointing to date. The best chance of cure is, therefore, by surgical excision of a small, early, peripheral tumour.

27. (a) T.
    (b) T.
    (c) F.
    (d) F.
    (e) T.
    Fractures of the neck and proximal shaft of femur occur commonly in elderly, osteoporotic females. Intracapsular fractures (subcapital and transcervical) risk avascular necrosis of the femoral head because the blood supply to the head is intraosseous at this level. The risk is particularly high in greatly displaced fractures and the best treatment in these cases is probably replacement of the femoral head (hemiarthroplasty). Undisplaced intracapsular fractures are usually treated by closed reduction followed by fixation with two crossed screws placed percutaneously. Extracapsular fractures (basal, neck, intratrochanteric, subtrochanteric) are commonly treated with a 'screw and plate' (e.g. dynamic hip screw). Total hip replacement is rarely indicated as the primary treatment for femoral neck fractures, but is a useful salvage procedure for complications such as non-union or acetabular damage caused by hemiarthroplasty.

28. (a) F.
    (b) F.
    (c) T.
    (d) F.
    (e) F.

    Rectal examination will fail to identify most prostatic carcinomas. Transrectal ultrasonography, especially if combined with measurement of prostate specific antigen, is more sensitive. There is no strong evidence that vasectomy pre-disposes men to risk of prostatic carcinoma. Prostatic tumours are discovered in a large proportion of men undergoing prostatectomy, but the significance is not clear. Phenoxybenzamine is an alpha blocker which may help in benign prostatic hypertrophy. Prostatic tumours may respond to hormone manipulation, castration, oestrogens or LHRH (luteinizing hormone release hormone) antagonists. Radical prostatectomy is rarely performed in the UK, but transurethral prostatectomy may be indicated for symptomatic relief of bladder outlet obstruction.

29. (a) F.
    (b) F.
    (c) T.
    (d) T.
    (e) F.

    The mainstay of treatment for severe acute pancreatitis is supportive and involves aggressive replacement of the extensive fluid losses intravenously. Multisystem failure, including respiratory failure and hypoxia, is a major complication and may be underestimated by clinical examination. Increased pulmonary permeability and subsequent oedema is the likely aetiology but should not prevent early aggressive fluid resuscitation. Fresh frozen plasma and proteolytic enzyme inhibitors (aprotinin) have been tried, but have failed to reduce mortality. Surgical intervention is reserved for complications such as pancreatic necrosis and abscess. Ultrasound scanning may suggest these diagnoses and may also reveal gallstones or dilated bile ducts. Should severe acute pancreatitis co-exist with a gallstone impacted in the ampulla of Vater, then endoscopic removal and sphincterotomy may reduce the risk of death.

30. (a) T.
    (b) F.
    (c) F.
    (d) T.
    (e) F.

A patient presenting with haematuria needs investigating to exclude a renal tract tumour and this entails an ultrasound scan of the upper renal tracts and bladder, or IVU, and cystoscopy to exclude early bladder tumours. Haematuria can be caused by infection, but infection can occur when there is other pathology in the urinary tract and so it cannot be assumed that a positive urine culture is the cause without excluding other pathology. Renal calculi usually cause haematuria, even if apparent only on testing. Despite investigation no cause will be found for an episode of haematuria in some patients who should be reviewed to make sure that an early tumour was not missed.

31. (a) T.
    (b) F.
    (c) F.
    (d) T.
    (e) T.

Colles' fracture of the distal radius commonly occurs in elderly patients following a fall onto an outstretched hand. The classic 'dinner fork' deformity results, which should be treated by closed manipulation under local, intravenous regional or general anaesthesia followed by plaster back slab. Redisplacement and malunion may occur resulting in an ugly appearance but usually an acceptable functional result, and internal fixation is not usually required. Nerve injuries are rare, but the median nerve is most at risk.

32. (a) F.
    (b) T.

(c) F.
(d) T.
(e) F.

A carcinoma is a malignant neoplasm arising from epithelium. Local invasion is a characteristic of malignancy, but early distant spread is more likely to be via lymphatics. Carcinomas usually form a firm mass which may ulcerate due to ischaemic necrosis of the centre. Sarcomas are malignant neoplasms of connective tissue. They tend to form soft masses which may compress surrounding structures, forming a false 'capsule'. They tend to metastasize early via the blood stream.

33. (a) T.
(b) F.
(c) T.
(d) F.
(e) T.

Scoliosis is a lateral curvature of the spine which is associated with rotation of the vertebral bodies. Detection can be difficult until obvious deformity becomes apparent which is more noticeable in the thoracic spine than the lumbar spine. Presentation for these reasons is often not until late childhood. The condition tends to progress until growth of the spine has ceased. After that further deterioration is much less rapid, so early detection and intervention to limit the condition should begin as early as possible.

Over 80% of patients with scoliosis have no apparent underlying cause. Hip problems such as untreated congenital dislocation resulting in leg shortening may result in compensatory scoliosis. Disc prolapse and developmental problems of the spine such as spina bifida are also associated with scoliosis. Neurological problems such as cerebral palsy or poliomyelitis or primary muscle disease may be associated with scoliosis.

Initial treatment is physiotherapy and spinal braces combined with regular review to assess the deformity which can be measured on X-ray. If the condition continues to progress, or interferes with other functions such as respiration, then surgical correction and fusion combined with some form of internal fixation such as a Harrington rod is required.

34. (a) F.
    (b) F.
    (c) F.
    (d) T.
    (e) F.
    Free gas will not be seen in 30% of cases, but care needs to be taken to exclude acute myocardial infarction and pancreatitis. Perforated duodenal ulcers are 4–5 times more common than gastric ulcers. Omental patches are associated with a higher ulcer recurrence rate than definitive operations such as truncal or highly selective vagotomy. However, depending on the experience of the surgeon and the condition of the patient, combined with H_2-receptor antagonists this is still a widely practised treatment. The ingestion of NSAIDs is not an indication for more definitive surgery. These patients are often elderly and there is evidence that H_2-receptor antagonists reduce the risk of perforation on NSAIDs. Perforation over 24 hours before concurrent medical illness and a pre-operative hypotension are factors associated with a higher mortality, although resuscitation must be adequate before surgery.

35. (a) T.
    (b) T.
    (c) F.
    (d) F.
    (e) T.
    Epidural anaesthesia is achieved by infusing local analgesics (e.g. bupivacaine) and/or opiates via a cannula placed in the extradural space of the spinal cord. It is particularly useful for operations on the lower limbs, especially in vascular surgery as the resulting vasodilatation reduces peripheral resistance and increases graft flow. There are obvious advantages in avoiding a general anaesthetic in someone with chronic lung disease, but epidural anaesthesia may be hazardous in patients with cardiac insufficiency,

particularly aortic stenosis, as cardiac output cannot rise to compensate for peripheral vasodilatation. The risk of epidural haematoma (which may lead to paraplegia) is obviously increased by anticoagulation.

36. (a) T.
    (b) F.
    (c) F.
    (d) T.
    (e) F.

The presentation of acute leg ischaemia is changing. Sudden occlusion of a normal artery due to emboli, often of cardiac origin (after myocardial infarction or due to an arrhythmia), is relatively less common and many patients present with a sudden thrombotic occlusion of an already diseased artery (acute on chronic presentation). These patients may have a previous history of claudication or arterial surgery, but it is often unclear from the history and angiography is usually required. Angiography allows planning of therapy and prevents inappropriate intervention such as an attempted balloon embolectomy in a diseased, thrombosed artery.

Thrombolytic agents (streptokinase or tissue plasminogen activator in the UK; urokinase in the USA) are increasingly being used in the treatment of acute ischaemia. Intravenous administration is associated with an unacceptably high systemic complication rate (e.g. intracranial bleeding). Intra-arterial administration of the drug directly into the clot by catheter is most commonly used, either by continuous low-dose infusion or more recently by high-dose bolus techniques which are more rapid.

Neuronal tissue is very sensitive to ischaemia and loss of sensation and motor function is one of the first indicators of severe ischaemia and precedes signs of muscle and skin damage. Unless the blood supply to the limb is rapidly restored tissue loss will occur. Usually this means surgical intervention, although the more rapid bolus thrombolytic techniques may be satisfactory. The priority is to re-establish blood supply to the leg, but placing the foot in dependency and increasing the patient's inspired oxygen, may marginally improve tissue perfusion as a temporary measure.

37. (a) F.
    (b) T.
    (c) T.
    (d) T.
    (e) T.

Following a burn injury there is a generalized increase in vascular endothelial permeability resulting in loss of fluid into the tissues which is maximal at 6–18 hours. This results in hypovolaemia and can cause respiratory failure secondary to pulmonary oedema. Loss of sensation is an indication of a full-thickness burn. There is a lowered resistance to staphylococcal and streptococcal infections and antibiotic prophylaxis is usually given. Care is needed, however, not to overadminister broad-spectrum antibiotics, as infection with resistant strains of *Staphylocossus* or *Pseudomonas* can be troublesome. Some units only give antibiotics for specific infections. Peptic ulcers (Curling's ulcer) may develop and prophylaxis is often given, but there is no strong evidence that H_2-receptor antagonists are effective.

38. (a) F.
    (b) T.
    (c) T.
    (d) F.
    (e) T.

An arteriovenous fistula is an abnormal communication between an artery and a vein bypassing the capillary bed. Resistance to blood flow through the fistula is less than through the normal circulation, so fistulas tend to enlarge with time and only rarely close spontaneously. As blood flow through the fistula rises, cardiac output increases to compensate. If flow is very high in a patient who is elderly or has heart disease, this may result in high-output cardiac failure. Ischaemia distal to the fistula due to steal may also occur.

Arteriovenous fistulas may be congenital in origin, although these lesions tend to be more complex and behave differently. Injury to an adjacent artery and vein, commonly by penetrating injuries (including surgery) but occasionally after blunt trauma, can result in a fistula and rarely diseased arteries may rupture into a vein (aortic aneurysm leaking into the inferior vena cava). Fistulas are also created to increase blood flow through a conduit or vein, e.g. for haemodialysis.

Surgical excision of arteriovenous fistulas can be difficult, incomplete and result in excessive blood loss. For large or complicated fistulas angiographic demonstration of the feeding and draining vessels is vital. In some cases it is possible to block these by selective catheter-directed embolization with material such as gelatin sponge or metal coils. More recently, Dacron-covered stents have been placed to occlude the fistula successfully.

39. (a) F.
    (b) F.
    (c) T.
    (d) T.
    (e) F.

Crush fractures of the vertebrae occur after transmission of force longitudinally across the vertebral body, as may occur in a fall from a height when the subject lands on their feet. If the bone is abnormal due to metastatic tumour or osteoporosis then the force of the injury may be minor and the fracture is pathological. Treatment is usually analgesia and rest. Crush fractures are generally stable, as the longitudinal ligaments are intact. Paraplegia is very uncommon, but can result from protrusion of the crushed vertebral body into the spinal canal. This is common in association with malignant deposits in the spine.

40. (a) F.
    (b) F.
    (c) T.
    (d) T.
    (e) T.

Superficial spreading melanomas may occur in benign naevae and spread horizontally (along the skin) before vertically (down into the skin). Nodular melanomas occur *de novo*, immediately spread vertically and thus carry a worse prognosis. Prognosis is related to depth or level of skin penetration and to extent of distant spread (clinical stage). For example, lesions less than 0.76 mm thick have rarely spread distantly, can be excised locally and carry an excellent prognosis, whereas melanomas greater than 1.5 mm thick are invariably associated with lymph node involvement and a poor 5-year survival (Breslow classification). An alternative classification concerns the level of skin penetration (Clark classification). For example, level I has not penetrated the epithelial basement membrane and carries a near 100% 5-year survival, but level V has extended through the skin into subcutaneous fat and is associated with a survival of less then 20%.

41. (a) T.
    (b) F.
    (c) F.
    (d) T.
    (e) F.

Papillary carcinoma of the thyroid may affect any age group but is commonest in early life. It carries an excellent prognosis and is usually effectively treated by total or subtotal thyroidectomy and then thyroxine to suppress thyroid stimulatory hormone, which may stimulate tumour growth. Follicular carcinoma carries a slightly worse prognosis and is likely to spread to lung and bone but secondary carcinomas may be treated by radio-iodine following total thyroidectomy. Anaplastic carcinoma affects older people and carries a very poor prognosis, but radiotherapy may provide some short-term relief.

42. (a) F.
    (b) F.
    (c) T.
    (d) F.
    (e) T.

The incidence of DVT depends on a number of factors including the age of the patient, the type of operation, the method of diagnosis and the use of prophylaxis. This can range from 80% for a total knee replacement to 30% for a pelvic operation, but overall is greater than 5%. The initiating events probably occur while the patient is on the operating table, although the DVT may not become clinically apparent for some time. Chronic venous insufficiency may occur due to venous valve damage or failure to recannulize the occluded veins, and this can result in venous ulceration. The DVTs may lead to pulmonary emboli, chronic venous insufficiency and varicose veins and so should be considered significant. Duplex ultrasound, especially if direction of flow is colour coded, is replacing venography as the first-line method of diagnosis of DVT.

43. (a) T.
    (b) F.
    (c) F.
    (d) T.
    (e) T.

Fracture dislocation usually follows forcible flexion combined with rotation of the spine resulting in fracture through the vertebral body and the posterior facet joints, tearing the posterior longitudinal ligament. This results in an unstable condition and the spinal cord may be injured at the time or during subsequent movement of the patient.

Between T10 and L1 the spinal canal contains both the spinal cord and the lumbar nerve roots which travel down to their respective foramina due to the disparity between the length of the bony vertebral column and the spinal cord. Above this level the canal contains only the cord and below only the nerve roots. Injury to the spinal cord may result in concussion only which, after a period of flaccid paralysis and sensory loss, recovers over the next few days. The anal reflex is served by the sacral roots and these will be below the level of injury. If the cord is transected, after a period of spinal shock, penile and anal reflexes return, but motor and sensory innervation supplied by the lumbar roots, is permanently lost. The nerve roots may also be injured alone, together with the cord at this level.

Treatment is to prevent neurological injury or to prevent further damage occurring. As the fracture is unstable the patient must be turned in one piece by experienced personnel. Stability can be maintained either by surgical fixation or by nursing the patient in a plaster cast. If the patient is paraplegic then specialized care is needed to prevent pressure sores, contractures and to manage the bladder and bowel. Failure to empty the bladder may result in overflow incontinence. In spinal units intermittent catheterization is usually undertaken to reduce the risk of infection, but often an indwelling catheter is used initially until the general condition of the patient is stable. Surgical decompression of the spinal cord is seldom of value and results in further instability.

44. (a) F.
    (b) F.
    (c) T.
    (d) F.
    (e) T.

Fractured ribs are suspected clinically by tenderness over a traumatized area and pain on inspiration. Crepitus or surgical emphysema suggests pneumothorax. This and other potential complications (haemothorax and damage to the intrathoracic structures) may be seen on a chest X-ray. It can be difficult to see rib fractures on X-ray, however, and the number of ribs fractured is usually underestimated. Strapping the chest restricts respiratory movements. Pain relief is better provided by systemic analgesics combined with intercostal nerve blocks. Young, fit people with isolated fractures do not require hospital admission, but elderly patients need admission for pain relief, physiotherapy and antibiotics to prevent pneumonia. Fracture of the first rib implies extreme traumatic force and damage to important structures such as the subclavian vessels or brachial plexus is a real risk.

45. (a) T.
    (b) T.
    (c) T.
    (d) F.
    (e) T.

The cervical spine is involved in approximately 25% of patients with RA. It may be asymptomatic, but often presents with painful restricted neck movements. Nerve root signs may be present. The atlantoaxial joint is commonly involved and can result in instability of the joint, exacerbated by neck flexion such as occurs during endotracheal intubation, when spinal cord injury may occur. X-rays of the cervical spine usually reveal the extent of the damage. Analgesics, anti-inflammatory drugs and rest in a cervical collar may be sufficient in many cases. Posterior fusion is occasionally required for progressive disease, especially if associated with neurological deficit.

46. (a) F.
    (b) T.
    (c) T.
    (d) T.
    (e) F.

Blunt injury in the loin may damage the kidney or renal artery, the ribs, spleen or liver. The ureter is unlikely to be injured due to its position in front of the psoas muscle alongside the vertebral column. In most cases a minor injury to the kidney will resolve and the haematuria will progressively lessen. An IVU should be obtained at the time of presentation because if intervention becomes necessary the presence of a contralateral kidney will be confirmed. Persistent or excessive bleeding requires surgical intervention to repair or remove the kidney. If possible, angiography is undertaken prior to this to identify the source of bleeding which can occasionally be stopped by therapeutic embolization. Secondary haemorrhage can occur 5–10 days later and other complications include hypertension due to renal artery damage, hydronephrosis and pseudocyst formation.

47. (a) F.
    (b) F.
    (c) F.
    (d) T.
    (e) F.
    The neutrophil count is raised in 95% of patients with acute appendicitis, and leucocytes can be found in the urine in the absence of a urinary-tract infection. Plain abdominal films are rarely helpful. Ultrasound may be helpful if a distended or oedematous appendix is seen, but often the exclusion of other pathology (e.g. ovarian cysts) is important. An appendix mass is usually treated with antibiotics and observation with appendicectomy at a later date. Surgery is undertaken if it fails to resolve, or as a planned intervention to avoid further treatment in the future.

48. (a) F.
    (b) F.
    (c) T.
    (d) F.
    (e) F.
    Ischaemic rest pain alone does not necessarily imply imminent limb loss and often fluctuates. If it persists and is associated with a low ankle systolic blood pressure (usually taken as <50 mmHg) limb loss is more likely without intervention and is termed critical limb ischaemia. Ischaemic rest pain is usually worse at night, as systemic blood pressure falls when the patient sleeps. The patient wakes with the pain and gets relief by hanging their leg over the bed, which marginally increases the perfusion of the foot. Patients with critical limb ischaemia tend to be elderly and do poorly after amputation so, wherever possible, arterial reconstruction should be undertaken. The majority of patients (over 90% in some series) are found to have disease of vessels suitable for bypass or angioplasty and can be offered treatment. Lumbar sympathectomy is often employed, but there is no objective evidence that it is of benefit by itself.

49. (a) F.
    (b) T.
    (c) F.
    (d) F.
    (e) T.

The earliest symptom is most frequently dysphagia and pain usually occurs late. The underlying pathology is degeneration of the cholinergic innervation of the distal two-thirds of the oesophagus which can occur at any age and is associated with an increased risk of malignancy. Treatment is either dilatation of the cardio-oesophageal sphincter or surgical incision of the muscle, leaving the mucosa intact (Heller myotomy).

50. (a) F.
    (b) T.
    (c) T.
    (d) T.
    (e) F.

Dislocation of the humeral head most commonly occurs anteriorly following a fall on an outstretched arm in the adult. Such an injury in the young results in a slipped humeral epiphysis, and in the elderly in a fracture of the neck of the humerus. Posterior dislocation is rare and may follow a direct impact to the front of the shoulder. Although the diagnosis may be apparent from the history and angular shape of the shoulder, the injury may be missed. If any doubt exists after an anteroposterior X-ray, a lateral view may be very helpful, showing the humeral head in front of the glenoid cavity.

Associated fractures and nerve injuries are relatively common. The circumflex nerve is the most commonly injured and supplies sensation to skin overlying the deltoid muscle and is also the motor supply to that muscle. Treatment is closed reduction and, although hand exercises are encouraged, shoulder movements are generally restricted for 3–4 weeks to allow healing of the joint capsule and to prevent recurrence.

Recurrent dislocation of the shoulder usually follows a traumatic dislocation. Physiotherapy may maintain the rotator cuff muscles, but surgical repair is required in most young adults (e.g. Putti–Platt or Bankart repair).

Answers to Paper 2

1. (a) T.
   (b) F.
   (c) T.
   (d) F.
   (e) T.
   Renal adenocarcinomas commonly present as a mass, with pain or haematuria. Although haematuria implies that the tumour has invaded the renal collecting system, it is still quite a frequent mode of presentation. Nephrectomy is the mainstay of treatment, although if the tumour is small and isolated to one pole a partial nephrectomy may be possible. The tumour may involve the inferior vena cava, but it is usually possible to remove it. The tumours are not radiosensitive.

2. (a) T.
   (b) F.
   (c) T.
   (d) F.
   (e) T.
   Reflux of urine into the ureters during micturition is a common finding in children investigated for urinary-tract infections. It may be demonstrated by ultrasound or an intravenous urogram, but is most reliably seen by a micturating cystogram. Reflux back-up to the renal pelvis, especially if associated with blunted calyces, risks renal scarring and subsequent renal failure. Lesser degrees of reflux appear to be relatively harmless. Over three-quarters of cases will resolve spontaneously and no treatment is necessary. Persistent bacteriuria is controlled by long-term low dose antibiotics, but severe reflux requires surgical intervention to reimplant the ureters into the bladder. Risks of renal scarring are rare over the age of 5 years.

3. (a) T.
   (b) F.
   (c) T.
   (d) F.
   (e) F.

   Prognosis of breast cancer is related to the size of the tumour, histological grade and extent of spread, including degree of axillary node involvement. Local control of the disease has a limited effect on survival because micrometastases are likely to have developed by the time of presentation. Local tumour excision and adjuvant radiotherapy are as effective as mastectomy in most cases. Survival is definitely improved by tamoxifen in women over 50 years of age (post-menopausal women) and possibly also in younger women. Adjuvant chemotherapy reduces mortality in younger women, whilst the role of oophorectomy (to induce 'menopause') is being investigated.

4. (a) F.
   (b) F.
   (c) F.
   (d) T.
   (e) T.

   Although symptoms usually begin in childhood, sometimes presentation may be delayed into adulthood. Laxatives are rarely effective. There is an absence of ganglion cells over a segment, usually originating in the rectosigmoid junction. The biopsy must be full thickness to establish that no ganglion cells are present. When the rectum distends the anus fails to relax.

5. (a) F.
   (b) T.
   (c) F.
   (d) F.
   (e) T.

   Adenocarcinoma of the pancreas is increasing in incidence and accounts for over 6000 deaths in the UK per year. Diagnosis may be delayed and simple imaging techniques may easily miss a 'hidden' retroperitoneal tumour. Computerized tomography scanning or magnetic resonance imaging are more helpful. The prognosis is very poor, with a 5-year survival of <5%. Pancreatic carcinoma is slightly more common in men than women. The exact cause is unknown, but there is an association with smoking, exposure to certain chemicals and diabetes.

6. (a) T.
   (b) F.
   (c) T.
   (d) T.
   (e) F.
   Supracondylar fracture of the humerus commonly occurs in children following a fall with the elbow flexed, pushing the distal fragment of the humerus posteriorly. The brachial artery may be injured or compressed by the distal humeral fragment, and absence of the radial pulse or tense tender forearm suggest a compartment syndrome requiring angiography and, if necessary, repair of the artery. Median and ulnar nerve injuries may also occur, but are usually due to neuropraxia and recover without direct intervention.
   Closed reduction with correction of the posterior displacement and rotation of the distal humerus is the first-line treatment. The triceps tendon anchors the fragment in position if the elbow is kept flexed after reduction with a collar and cuff and plaster back slab. Open reduction can cause damage to the epiphyses and is avoided unless adequate closed reduction is not possible. Some degree of correction of anterior/posterior angulation will correct with bone remodelling, but rotation and lateral tilt will leave an ugly restricted elbow and reduction must be satisfactory.

7. (a) T.
   (b) T.
   (c) T.
   (d) F.
   (e) F.
   Leucoplakia is a pre-cancerous condition and may lead to

cancer of the tongue. Smoking and poor oral hygiene also pre-dispose to this tumour which is generally a squamous cell carcinoma. Cancer of the tongue often presents as an ulcer on the tip or side of the tongue, but when it arises on the posterior part it often presents late and so carries a worse prognosis. Approximately half of patients will have palpable lymph nodes at presentation. Treatment is usually surgical resection of the tumour (partial or total glossectomy), block dissection of the neck if lymph nodes are involved followed by radiotherapy. Local radiation with iodine-192 may be used for early lesions.

8. (a) T.
   (b) F.
   (c) F.
   (d) T.
   (e) F.

In a healthy adult male 60% of body weight is water (less in females and the elderly). Thus about 40 litres of water is divided between circulating volume (3 litres), interstitial fluid (12 litres) (together compromising extracellular fluid), and intracellular fluid (25 litres). Extracellular fluid is rich in sodium (140 mmol/l) and poor in potassium (4–4.5 mmol/l) with chloride as the predominant anion. Intracellular fluid contains 150 mmol/l of potassium, much less sodium (10 mmol/l) and substantial quantities of phosphate, sulphate and protein as anions.

9. (a) T.
   (b) F.
   (c) T.
   (d) T.
   (e) F.

It is estimated that 3–5% of cases of hypertension are due to atheromatous narrowing of the renal artery. This results in reduced renal perfusion pressure with subsequent increased renin/angiotensin activity, causing hypertension. Reduced renal perfusion may result in impaired renal function, but again it is unclear in how many patients with renal failure the cause is underlying renal artery disease.

Numerous cases of improved renal function following treatment of the renal artery disease have been reported. Occasionally a bruit due to a stenosed renal artery may be audible in the epigastrium or flank. Diagnosis is difficult and involves duplex ultrasound, isotope renography and angiography.

Lesions in the stem of the renal artery are amenable to angioplasty. The lesion often encroaches into the aorta, and surgery is then the best option. Bypass grafts from the aorta, often combined with aortic reconstruction, give good results, but are major undertakings in patients who are often elderly and unfit. Autotransplantation can be undertaken but, recently, interest in using the splenic artery on the left or the hepatic artery on the right to improve the renal perfusion has increased. This is not such a major operation from the patient's perspective. If the kidney is small, shrunken and poorly functioning and the patient has uncontrolled hypertension, nephrectomy may be the only option.

10. (a) T.
    (b) T.
    (c) F.
    (d) F.
    (e) F.

This is a controversial area as many reports of prophylaxis are too small to show benefit. Aspirin has recently been suggested by meta-analysis to have a small but significant effect on the incidence of DVT. Although more major surgery carries a greater risk of DVT, the operating time itself has not been proved to relate to the risk of DVT. Compression stockings do reduce the risk of DVT but this has not been shown to reduce the risk of pulmonary emboli. The standard-dose oestrogen contraceptive pill has been shown to increase the risk of DVT about six-fold. The risk with the low-dose pill is less clear, but it appears to increase the risk about two-fold and the effects of taking it take 6 weeks to wear off. No study has even been undertaken to determine if there is any benefit in stopping the low-dose pill prior to surgery. Subcutaneous heparin

(5000 units, 2 or 3 times daily) has been shown in a multicentre trial and a meta-analysis to reduce post-operative DVT and pulmonary emboli. Some surgeons do not accept these results. DVTs begin whilst the patient is on the operating table, so to have any protective effect standard unfractionated heparin must be given 4–6 hours prior to surgery to allow it to work before the clotting mechanisms are activated by the operation.

11. (a) T.
    (b) F.
    (c) T.
    (d) T.
    (e) F.

A subdural empyema is a collection of pus beneath the dura which has often spread from a paranasal sinus or middle-ear infection. It can also occur after trauma and surgery. Streptococci and staphylococci are often isolated. The patients are usually very unwell, level of consciousness may be depressed, and CT scan may confirm the diagnosis. Treatment involves antibiotics, treatment of the underlying cause (e.g. drainage of the sinuses) and removal and culture of the pus. As pus may be diffusely spread in the subdural space, multiple burr holes and irrigation or removal of areas of the skull may be required to clear it adequately.

12. (a) T.
    (b) F.
    (c) F.
    (d) F.
    (e) T.

Inguinal hernias in children result from failure of the processus vaginalis to close. Often, the hernia cannot be demonstrated but a precise history from the mother (especially if combined with the sac being palpated by rolling the cord over the pubic tubercle) is enough to make the diagnosis. Spontaneous closure of a processus vaginalis that is open enough to admit a loop of bowel is unlikely, and elective inguinal herniotomy (ligation of the processus vaginalis at the deep ring) is the best treatment. Children seen with painful, irreducible hernias should be treated by sedation and leg elevation followed by normal reduction of the hernia. Herniotomy is then performed 48 hours later when oedema has settled. If strangulation is suspected, then urgent surgical intervention is required.

13. (a) F.
    (b) T.
    (c) F.
    (d) T.
    (e) F.

Fibroadenomas are seen most commonly in women under 30 years, but may also occur in older women. The diagnosis is often made clinically and mammography is unnecessary and unhelpful. Fine-needle aspiration cytology is useful, especially in older women, and to exclude a simple cyst. Fibroadenomas are classically firm, mobile, asymptomatic lumps ('breast mice'). Traditional treatment recommended is simple excision and most women request that the lump is removed. However, some surgeons believe that a classical fibroadenoma in a young woman may be safely left *in situ* if it has not changed in size over a few months.

14. (a) T.
    (b) F.
    (c) T.
    (d) T.
    (e) F.

Fractures of the mandible are common and usually due to trauma, frequently in young males. The fracture site is nearly always in communication with the oral cavity and so it is assumed that the fracture is compound and antibiotics are given. The associated soft-tissue swelling may be extensive and any bony deformity may be missed. Any clinical suspicion of a fracture, such as pain or inability to open the mouth, crepitus, soft tissue swelling or areas of sensory loss (due to associated nerve damage, especially the inferior dental nerve), require careful X-ray examination.

Treatment is reduction and fixation. This may be achieved by dental wiring, but often requires internal fixation with a plate.

15. (a) F.
    (b) F.
    (c) T.
    (d) T.
    (e) F.

Radical surgery is reserved for those lesions that fail to respond to radiotherapy. The role of chemotherapy is still being evaluated. Spread to the inguinal lymph nodes is frequent, and these areas are usually included in the radiotherapy fields. 50% of patients have evidence of previous infection with human papilloma virus and presentation is usually with pain, bleeding or a lump.

16. (a) T.
    (b) F.
    (c) T.
    (d) T.
    (e) F.

Acute sinusitis results from secondary bacterial infection associated with an upper-respiratory-tract infection or, rarely, a fracture into the sinus. Dental disease can cause sinus infection due to the close proximity of the roots of the upper molars and the floor of the maxillary sinus. Diagnosis is usually made on clinical features: pyrexia, facial pain and nasal congestion. Opacity of the sinus may be apparent on X-ray. Treatment is with analgesics, antibiotics and nasal decongestants. Drainage of the maxillary sinus via the inferior meatus can be carried out if the condition does not respond to therapy; formal surgical drainage is only rarely undertaken. Complications of acute sinusitis include osteomyelitis, meningitis and intracranial abscess formation, orbital cellulitis and sagittal sinus thrombosis.

17. (a) F.
    (b) T.

(c) F.
(d) F.
(e) T.

Lipomas may be found in any body tissue ('the ubiquitous tumour'), but are most commonly seen in subcutaneous fat. They are usually lobulated, localized, encapsulated tumours that feel soft and fluctuant and are composed of normal-looking fat cells. Treatment is by surgical excision and is indicated for symptoms (e.g. pain) or cosmesis. Lipomas may be multiple. Dercum's disease (adipose dolorosa) describes multiple, diffuse, tender lipomas and is rare. Malignant potential is very low.

18. (a) F.
    (b) T.
    (c) F.
    (d) T.
    (e) T.

The state of body fluids is a result of a balance between intake and loss. The average daily intake of water is 3 litres: 2 litres are lost in urine and 1 litre from the skin and lungs. ADH is released from the posterior lobe of the pituitary gland, usually in response to hypertonicity or hypovolaemia, and results in water retention and concentrated urine. Decreased circulating blood volume produces a dramatic response, with renin release from the juxtaglomerular apparatus in the kidney, which results in increased renal sodium (and thus water) reabsorption. Other mechanisms (local renal autoregulation and catecholamines) are also involved in sodium and water metabolism, and stimuli such as pain and tissue trauma also initiate a water-retaining response.

19. (a) F.
    (b) F.
    (c) T.
    (d) T.
    (e) F.

5% dextrose is merely a convenient way of providing water in an isotonic solution. Isotonic (normal) saline contains

154 mmol/l of sodium and an equal concentration of chloride which is, therefore, higher than the concentration in plasma. A healthy adult requires (approximately) 2 litres of water and 500 ml of saline to replace losses, but in ill or post-operative patients these requirements may vary tremendously. A high temperature increases sweating and also fluid-intake requirements.

20. (a) F.
    (b) F.
    (c) F.
    (d) T.
    (e) T.

It is not possible to predict the chances of a patient with simple varicose veins subsequently developing venous ulcers, nor is there evidence that prophylactic surgical intervention will reduce this risk. Varicose veins then should be treated on their own merits at the time of presentation.

The majority of patients have simple, superficial venous incompetence. The overall results of 'simple' varicose vein surgery are disappointing, with over 30% of patients getting significant recurrences over 10 years. It might be argued that better pre-operative investigation would allow directed surgical intervention and produce better results. Many units do this, but tend to rely on non-invasive tests such as simple ultrasound and, more recently, duplex ultrasound and colour-coded ultrasound which is replacing venography. LSI can be detected with simple tests such as the Trendelenburg test (although duplex ultrasound is probably more accurate). SSI is much more difficult to determine and duplex ultrasound is the most reliable method. Missed SSI is a major cause of 'recurrent' varicose veins. Investigation of the deep venous system is vital prior to superficial venous surgery if the patient has a history of deep vein thrombosis, significant trauma to the leg or limb swelling.

A number of surgical techniques are used to disconnect the incompetent superficial veins from the deep veins. 'Stripping' the LSV to the ankle is not widely practised now. Often the LSV is not itself varicose and the calf perforators and tributaries are left intact; the procedure is associated with morbidity and the LSV may be needed as an arterial bypass conduit in the future. Stripping the LSV to the knee is more commonly performed in an attempt to remove the mid-thigh perforator which is difficult to localize clinically and is another cause of 'recurrence'. The answer probably lies in better localization of the incompetent superficial veins using non-invasive techniques prior to surgery.

21. (a) T.
    (b) F.
    (c) F.
    (d) F.
    (e) T.

FAP is inherited through an autosomal dominant gene, but 25% of patients will be new mutations. Patients usually present in early adulthood and are often asymptomatic. Malignant transformation nearly always occurs over 10 years. A number of extracolonic manifestations have been noted, including epidermoid cysts, fibrous tumours, osteomas and congenital hypertrophy of the retinal pigmented epithelium (CHRPEs). CHRPEs is highly specific for FAP and is present before polyps occur.

22. (a) T.
    (b) F.
    (c) F.
    (d) T.
    (e) F.

Tumours of the maxillary antrum are mostly squamous cell carcinomas, rarely metastasize and present late with symptoms related to local invasion. These include nasal obstruction, dental or facial pain or proptosis due to orbital involvement. CT scans or magnetic resonance imaging are particularly valuable in defining the extent of the disease. Following biopsy, treatment is usually surgical resection of the tumour via a palatal fenestration followed by radiotherapy, or radiotherapy alone if the tumour is advanced.

23. (a) T.
    (b) F.
    (c) F.
    (d) T.
    (e) F.

The exact cause of varicose ulcers remains unclear. Venous incompetence results in increased venous pressure resulting in extravasation of white (WBC) and red (RBC) blood cells and plasma proteins such as fibrinogen into the tissues. This causes tissue damage, the WBCs become activated producing further damage. Fibrin is formed and it is suggested that this forms a barrier to perfusion between the nutrient blood vessels and the epidermis (fibrin cuff theory). The result is breakdown of the epidermis and ulcer formation, beginning usually over the medial aspect of the ankle.

Elevation and compression will reduce the venous pressure, and with adequate local treatment the ulcer will heal in over 60% of patients. This is time-consuming and the ulcer tends to recur unless the underlying problem is addressed.

Bacteria can be cultured from most ulcers, but are usually commensals and require no specific treatment. Overt infection with signs of systemic spread (redness, pain, lymphangitis, or pyrexia) requires appropriate systemic antibiotic therapy. There is no role for topical antibiotics.

24. (a) T.
    (b) T.
    (c) F.
    (d) F.
    (e) T.

Pain originating in the hip may be referred to the knee due to the close proximity of the obturator nerve to the hip joint capsule. In the patient complaining of knee pain in whom examination of that joint is normal, hip pathology should be considered. Pain and joint stiffness are often worse first thing in the morning (early morning stiffness) or after periods of immobility due to other conditions.

Pain, however, may persist and can continue even at night when the patient is non-weight bearing.

X-ray appearances of osteoarthritis are loss of joint space, subarticular sclerosis, cyst formation and osteophytes. First-line treatment is analgesia, anti-inflammatory drugs, weight loss, etc. If this is not adequate, osteotomy may be beneficial especially in the younger patient. The mode of action of osteotomy is unclear, but redistribution of the weight-bearing area of the joint combined with transection of the blood vessels and nerves of the periosteum seem to reduce pain effectively. Total hip arthroplasty is usually best avoided in younger patients and is performed in the more elderly and when gross joint destruction has occurred. Fusion of the hip, arthrodesis is necessary in some situations, e.g. after infection of a prosthetic hip. In younger patients who have good movements of the lumbar spine mobility is surprisingly good. In patients with widespread joint destruction arthrodesis usually results in marked loss of function.

25. (a) T.
    (b) F.
    (c) T.
    (d) T.
    (e) T.

Renal stones are relatively common and, in many patients, no cause will be found. It is important to exclude abnormalities of calcium metabolism (in particular hyperparathyroidism) and serum calcium and 24-hour calcium excretion should be checked. Stones may form in association with other abnormalities in the renal tract, including tumours. These should be excluded. If no specific cause is found, increasing fluid intake may reduce the chance of further stone formation.

26. (a) T.
    (b) F.
    (c) F.

(d) F.
(e) T.

The absence of a testicle from the scrotum may be due to retractile testis (strong cremasteric reflex), ectopic testicle (descended to an abnormal position), or incomplete descent (or atrophy due to intracanalicular torsion or failure to develop).

Testicles fail to descend properly because they are imperfectly formed (dyspastic), and are associated with an increased risk of malignant change. This risk is not reduced by orchidopexy, but such a change is more obvious at an early stage. The time at which to bring an incompletely descended testicle down to the scrotum remains controversial, but there is no strong evidence to suggest that early orchidopexy is advantageous. Operation before the child reaches school age seems appropriate.

Retractile (not incompletely descended) testicles are palpable in the scrotum at birth, but as the cremaster muscle develops may be difficult to feel at the age of 2 years. Puberty ensures that proper descent occurs eventually.

Retractile testicles may be milked down into the scrotum by gentle palpation. This is best performed with warm hands with the child squatting or lying with legs parted and flexed.

Most incompletely descended testicles are impalpable, either lost in the suprapubic fat pad, in the inguinal canal or, occasionally, intra-abdominal (seen on laparoscopy).

27. (a) T.
    (b) T.
    (c) F.
    (d) T.
    (e) F.

Breast pain is a common symptom, usually affecting women in their early to mid-40s. It is often cyclical with increased pain before menstruation and associated with fibrocystic change or breast nodularity. Symptoms may persist for weeks or years but usually disappear after menopause, though HRT may cause recurrence.

Carcinoma uncommonly presents with pain and women presenting with cyclical mastalgia are extremely unlikely to have breast cancer. The aetiology is unclear, but EFA deficiencies have been documented. Treatment includes reassurance about breast cancer, a good support bra and analgesics if necessary. Evening primrose oil contains EFA γ-linoleic acid (GLA), and has proved helpful in some women. GLA preparations are now available on prescription. The antioestrogens danazol and tamoxifen are sometimes used in severe cases (although tamoxifen is not licensed for this use in the UK).

28. (a) F.
    (b) T.
    (c) T.
    (d) T.
    (e) T.

Most adenomas are found incidentally during investigation for other purposes, are asymptomatic and often occur in association with other adenomas. Occasionally they can bleed, prolapse through the anus or cause intussusception. Some polyps secrete large volumes of mucus and result in diarrhoea and hypokalaemia. Adenomas are pre-malignant but the transformation rate is low and is related to histological type (villous adenomas are more likely to become malignant than are tubular adenomas) and increasing size. Further adenomas may develop, and colonoscopy is usually undertaken every 3–5 years.

29. (a) T.
    (b) T.
    (c) T.
    (d) F.
    (e) F.

Indications for THA include pain and stiffness from joint destruction due to osteoarthritis, rheumatoid arthritis, trauma, avascular necrosis or damage resulting from congenital abnormalities of the hip. Previous arthrodesis can also be converted into a THA.

Local complications include infection, which can occur

in up to 1% of patients without antibiotics. Meticulous surgical technique and laminar flow tents over the operating field have reduced infection rates. Antibiotics have also been shown to lower rates of infection and, if used for short periods (1–3 doses), are not associated with the development of resistant organisms. Bleeding, damage to surrounding structures such as nerves, fracture of the shaft of the femur or poor placement of the acetabulum can also occur. Loosening of the prosthesis may occur and can be seen on X-ray. In some patients this results in pain and requires revision. Early dislocation is initially treated by reduction and traction to allow healing. If it continues to occur it may be due to poor placement of the prosthesis, and revision will be required.

General complications include DVT, chest infections, myocardial infarction and, rarely, reactions to the cement used resulting in hypotension. DVT is particularly common, occurring in up to 30–50% of patients. Prophylaxis with heparin reduces the risk, but is associated with increased risk of bleeding complications, which may result in infection of the prosthesis. For this reason the role of heparin remains controversial. Low-molecular-weight heparins may have less risk of bleeding complications but with the same efficacy in reducing DVT, and are being assessed. Dextran infusions, compression stockings and pneumatic boots are used by some surgeons.

30. (a) F.
    (b) F.
    (c) F.
    (d) F.
    (e) T.

Graduated compression stockings may be successfully used for the long-term treatment of patients who do not wish to undergo, or are unfit for, surgery. These must be properly fitted and exert adequate compression in a graduated fashion (e.g. 30 mmHg at ankle, 15 mmHg above the knee) to be of value. Injection sclerotherapy can be used successfully to treat primary varicose veins. Recurrence can be a problem especially when marked saphenofemoral incompetence (SFI) is present and many surgeons deal with the SFI surgically and inject the remaining calf veins at a subsequent visit.

Deep venous reflux is usually due to previous damage to the valves of the deep veins and saphenofemoral ligation will not help. Patients with deep venous problems must be identified as they will not usually benefit from superficial venous surgery and may be made considerably worse. A history of deep vein thrombosis or limb trauma, marked limb swelling or a bursting pain on walking (venous claudication) should prompt duplex ultrasound or venography. Arterial disease is also very common and any suggestion of arterial insufficiency needs further investigation. If ankle pulses cannot be felt, the ankle systolic blood pressure should be measured. Compression therapy may further compromise the arterial circulation and venous surgery may result in the failure of incisions to heal or at the least the removal of a potential bypass conduit.

Varicose veins, particularly below the knee, may be removed through small 2–3 mm incisions by traction or by using small hooks. This leaves an acceptable cosmetic result.

31. (a) F.
    (b) F.
    (c) F.
    (d) F.
    (e) T.

Radical surgery carries a high mortality (up to 25%) and is still associated with a 5-year survival rate of less than 5%. The role of such procedures is controversial, but they should only be undertaken in selected patients. The mainstay of treatment is to relieve jaundice and control pain (palliation). Endoscopic biliary stenting is effective and may avoid the need for bypass surgery. CEA is raised in 80% of patients and falls following resection, not being specific to liver secondaries. Coeliac axis blockade may be effective in controlling pain due to invasion of the nerve plexus. Radiotherapy may find a place as an adjunct to surgery. Chemotherapy has been used in a small number of patients who are potentially 'curable', but it is generally ineffective.

32. (a) T.
    (b) T.
    (c) F.
    (d) T.
    (e) T.

Pneumothorax may occur secondary to trauma or tuberculosis, or spontaneously. Risk factors for the development of spontaneous pneumothorax are congenital alveolar wall defects, bullae resulting from chronic bronchitis, emphysema, lung cysts or alveolar hyperinflation secondary to positive-pressure ventilation. Presentation is as above and the diagnosis is usually confirmed by chest X-ray. Tension pneumothorax (caused by a valvular tear in the lung), however, is a genuine emergency and a cannula should be inserted immediately to relieve tension, followed by tube drainage, without waiting for an X-ray.

Treatment of a small, asymptomatic pneumothorax in a fit person may be conservative or simple aspiration may suffice. Larger pneumothoraces or dyspnoea are an indication for insertion of a tube drain.

Recurrent pneumothorax may be treated by procedures that cause adhesion between the lung and chest wall, such as talc insufflation via a thoracoscope.

33. (a) T.
    (b) F.
    (c) T.
    (d) F.
    (e) T.

Diabetes is a definite risk factor increasing the possibility of death from anaesthesia and major surgery. Risk of wound infection is also increased, especially in elderly, poorly controlled diabetics. Insulin-controlled diabetics should be converted to a 'sliding-scale' of insulin or a dextrose/insulin drip until they are back on their usual diet. Oral hypoglycaemics are not usually given pre-operatively due to the risk of hypoglycaemia. Blood sugar is monitored regularly and insulin given as required. Tablets are restarted on return to diet.

34. (a) T.
    (b) F.
    (c) F.
    (d) F.
    (e) T.
    Indications for tonsillectomy are debatable, but generally it is only undertaken if attacks of tonsillitis are frequent and causing a lot of discomfort. Local spread of the infection into the peritonsillar tissues can result in an abscess (quinsy) which results in pain on opening the mouth (trismus) and pain on swallowing. Treatment of this complication is by antibiotics and drainage followed by elective tonsillectomy. Tonsillectomy should not be undertaken in the presence of active infection which should be allowed to resolve completely first. Children with cleft palate may have incompetence of their nasopharyngeal sphincter even after repair of the palate. Scarring after tonsillectomy may make this worse, which adversely affects speech.

35. (a) F.
    (b) F.
    (c) F.
    (d) F.
    (e) T.
    Local analgesic infiltration anaesthesia is very useful for a wide range of minor surgical procedures. It is safe, but not entirely without hazard. Injection of too high a dose may result in serious neurological or cardiovascular complications, so the surgeon must be aware of the maximum safe doses. Bupivacaine is effective as a long-acting analgesic, but prilocaine has less systemic toxicity. A vasoconstrictor such as adrenaline reduces systemic spread and allows larger doses to be given, but they should not be used around end arteries (e.g. digits or penis) as they could

produce distal ischaemia and gangrene. Commercially available preparations of local anaesthetic are often more concentrated than is needed for simple infiltration anaesthesia, and the weakest solution (e.g. 1% lignocaine, 0.25% bupivacaine) is adequate. Full effect may take some minutes. Intravenous diazepam reduces patient anxiety and lowers the potential risk of convulsions, but should be used cautiously.

36. (a) T.
    (b) F.
    (c) T.
    (d) F.
    (e) T.

In FAP nearly all patients develop malignant transformation within 10 years of onset. There is evidence of an inherited risk of colorectal cancer in some families other than those affected by FAP. Some individuals have hereditary non-polyposis colon cancer, an autosomal dominant condition, present in up to 5% of patients with colon cancer. Long-standing active ulcerative colitis carries a significant risk of malignant transformation. The same applies to a lesser extent for Crohn's disease. Other risk factors include patients who previously had implantation of their ureter into the sigmoid colon for urinary diversion. The risk of colorectal cancer after cholecystectomy remains controversial. Diverticular disease and angiodysplasia do not increase the risk of colorectal malignancy.

37. (a) F.
    (b) T.
    (c) F.
    (d) F.
    (e) T.

Bleeding from diverticula may be massive but usually settles without surgical intervention. Complications of diverticular disease include haemorrhage, inflammation, perforation, stricture and fistula formation, most commonly into the bladder, but occasionally the vagina, causing persistent urinary-tract infection and pneumonia.

Bowel obstruction may occur due to an inflammatory mass or stricture formation. There is no increased risk of malignancy with diverticular disease, although the differential diagnosis may be difficult. Diverticula can occur elsewhere in the gut but are not associated with large-bowel diverticula.

38. (a) F.
    (b) F.
    (c) F.
    (d) T.
    (e) T.
    Bone metastases usually result from haematogenous spread. Sites commonly affected are vertebrae, pelvis, ribs, skull and upper humerus or femur. Breast (35%) and prostate (30%) are the most likely primaries, followed by lung, kidney and thyroid. Bone secondaries usually appear osteolytic but may be osteosclerotic, especially prostatic metastases. Bone tumours may be demonstrated by plain X-rays but isotope bone scanning is more sensitive and may also reveal unsuspected metastases at other sites. Pain may be controlled by anti-inflammatory and opiate analgesics, but radiotherapy is more effective and also reduces tumour mass. Radiotherapy causes osteolysis, however, and may therefore be complicated by pathological fractures. Radiotherapy may be preceded by internal fixation to avoid this. Established pathological fractures are most effectively managed by internal fixation (e.g. intramedullary nail) as it allows early mobilization and controls pain.

39. (a) F.
    (b) T.
    (c) T.
    (d) F.
    (e) F.
    Persistent hoarseness in anyone over the age of 40 years is presumed to be carcinoma of the larynx until proven otherwise. Laryngitis can cause hoarseness but is usually short lived and associated with systemic signs of infection.

Pain in the ear suggests glossopharyngeal nerve irritation and can be due to invasion by tumour. Overuse/misuse of the voice and benign nodules and polyps of the vocal chords can also cause hoarseness, but this is relatively uncommon and the diagnosis should always be supported by laryngoscopy. Carcinoma of the bronchus can invade the recurrent laryngeal nerve and present as hoarseness, so a chest X-ray should be obtained.

40. (a) F.
    (b) F.
    (c) T.
    (d) T.
    (e) T.

The peak age of presentation of these tumours is in the teens. A second peak occurs in the 60–70s when the malignant transformation has occurred in pre-existing Paget's disease. The tumours commonly affect the metaphyses of long bones around the knee, and the patient may present with a painful, hot swollen knee which may initially be mistaken for osteomyelitis, trauma or a benign tumour. The diagnosis may be made on X-ray, although magnetic resonance imaging is especially good at delineating the tumour, and biopsy. Treatment consists of staging the disease. Blood-borne metastases are common and especially affect the lungs. Removal of the primary tumour by amputation or, increasingly, combined with reconstruction of the limb using prosthetic implants, is followed by chemotherapy.

41. (a) F.
    (b) F.
    (c) T.
    (d) F.
    (e) T.

Paraoesophageal hernia describes herniation of the fundus of the stomach through the diaphragmatic hiatus and into the chest, *alongside* a normally placed oesophagus. Such 'rolling' hernias are not normally associated with reflux, unlike 'sliding' hernias when the upper stomach is displaced into the thorax with the gastro-oesophageal junction. Incidence increases with age as the hiatus becomes lax. Symptoms are mechanical – attacks of pain and post-prandial vomiting. A gastric ulcer may form in the hernia and cause bleeding and anaemia. Intermittent thoracic incarceration may exacerbate symptoms and strangulation is a risk. It is usually prudent, therefore, to repair paraoesophageal hernias electively after confirmation of the diagnosis by barium meal (endoscopy may be confusing).

42. (a) T.
    (b) T.
    (c) F.
    (d) F.
    (e) T.

Injuries to the medial meniscus generally occur due to rotation forces acting on a flexed knee. Cysts and congenital abnormalities can pre-dispose to meniscal injury, but are more common in the lateral cartilage. With increasing age the meniscus becomes less elastic and may suffer injury following a relatively minor injury. The medial meniscus is avascular and so a haemarthrosis will only occur if the peripheral part is torn. Initially, locking of the knee may occur and the torn segment of cartilage may block knee extension. Diagnosis is usually made on clinical grounds, but arthroscopy may be needed if there is uncertainty. It is also possible to remove the torn segment or the whole meniscus using the arthroscope treating the patient at the same time. Injury to the meniscus is, however, associated with a greater risk of secondary osteoarthritis.

43. (a) F.
    (b) F.
    (c) T.
    (d) F.
    (e) T.

Septic shock describes a syndrome that may result from bacterial endotoxaemia (classically from Gram-negative organisms in the gut) or severe inflammatory reactions following major trauma or surgery. Initially, there is a hyperdynamic circulation with a high CVP and warm extremities due to increased cardiac output and vasodilatation, though later myocardial depression may result and this requires inotropic support. Broad-spectrum intravenous antibiotics should be started immediately after blood and other relevant cultures have been sent for analysis. Toxins and inflammatory mediators result in increased pulmonary permeability and adult respiratory distress syndrome, requiring ventilation.

44. (a) T.
    (b) F.
    (c) F.
    (d) F.
    (e) F.

Heparin is commenced on diagnosis. Most commonly, a bolus is followed by a continuous intravenous infusion. The bolus dose can be calculated on a body weight basis (70 units/kg body weight), but the subsequent rate of infusion is variable and must be titrated carefully against the activated partial thromboplastin time (APTT) which should be 2–3 times greater than the control value. Heparin can be given subcutaneously for the treatment of DVT; doses are controlled by APTT and are given 3 times a day. The total daily dose is similar to the intravenous route and is much greater than 5000 units, which is the dose used for thromboprophylaxis.

The optimum duration of heparin therapy, which determines when oral anticoagulation is commenced, is controversial and many clinicians feel that it should be 10 days. Recent evidence suggests that the complication and thromboembolic recurrence rate is no different if oral anticoagulation is commenced within a day of diagnosis. Most clinicians commence warfarin after 3–4 days with 2–3 days combined treatment until warfarin therapy is satisfactory. Clinical signs are not reliable and are not generally a factor in deciding when to commence oral anticoagulation. Massive thrombosis with marked limb swelling is an exception and treatment has to be tailored to the individual situation.

Uncontrolled reports of thrombolysis in selected patients with extensive DVT are encouraging. An initial bolus dose is followed by a continuous infusion. At present this therapy is still very much under evaluation and should not be used routinely.

45. (a) T.
    (b) F.
    (c) F.
    (d) T.
    (e) F.

Injuries to the urethra are commonly associated with fractures of the pelvis. The initial displacement of the pelvic ring at the time of injury and the attachments of the prostate and bulbar urethra usually cause rupture or tearing of the membraneous urethra. Fresh blood at the external meatus should alert the clinician to this possibility. The bladder needs to be catheterized to monitor urine output during resuscitation and to prevent extravasation of urine into the injured perineum. Some experienced urologists advocate the attempted passage of a soft urethral catheter. In practice, if the patient has other serious injuries and the expertise is not immediately available, it is better to place a suprapubic catheter. Repair of the urethra can then be undertaken when the condition of the patient allows, which might be over a week later.

46. (a) F.
    (b) T.
    (c) F.
    (d) T.
    (e) T.

Pain and restriction of hip movement in children (irritable hip) is most commonly caused by a supposed transient synovitis, occasionally preceded by a history of minor trauma or overuse. Investigations and X-rays are normal and the child improves with rest. However, the importance lies in detecting other more serious conditions which, in general, are made worse with use.

Perthes' disease is a condition which affects the blood supply to the femoral head and can result in avascular necrosis. Initial presentation is usually between 5 and 10 years of age and is more common in boys, but the condition often episodically progresses over a number of years. Initial investigations may appear normal. Early X-ray changes include increased joint space and granularity of the femoral head followed by flattening as further destruction occurs. Isotope bone scan may show areas of avascular bone. Treatment consists of immobilization of the hip either by traction in bed or by abducting the hip with a splint to increase the angle of 'containment' of the hip joint. Some surgeons undertake an osteotomy in order to try to achieve this.

The epiphyseal plate at the upper end of the femur may slip. More common in overweight boys around puberty, it may present between 10 and 15 years of age. The condition can be recognized on X-ray. If there is a minor displacement of the epiphysis further displacement is prevented by placing three pins along the femoral neck into the epiphysis. If displacement is marked then either open reduction (which is associated with a high risk of avascular necrosis) or fixation of the epiphysis with a subsequent osteotomy to correct deformity resulting from growth abnormalities is performed.

Septic arthritis is usually associated with systemic signs of infection. The infection is most often blood borne from another focus. Aspiration of the joint will confirm the diagnosis and allow appropriate antibiotic therapy. Rheumatoid arthritis may present in childhood. Other joints may be involved, but occasionally a monoarthritis occurs. Osteoarthritis may occur secondary to CDH, but the presentation is usually in middle age.

47. (a) F.
    (b) T.
    (c) F.

(d) T.
(e) F.

In UC the inflammatory process is limited to the mucosa and so fistulas rarely form. The inflamed mucosa develops ulcers and, if severe, this gives the appearance of polyps (hence pseudopolyps) on barium enema (compare with cobblestoning and deep 'rose-thorn' ulcers in Crohn's disease). Orosomucoid (α_1-acid glycoprotein) is a non-specific acute-phase protein made in the liver. The level may be raised if the disease is active, but it must be interpreted together with other criteria and clinical features. Early toxic dilatation may be treated with steroids, but usually it is severe and total colectomy is required. UC usually begins in the rectum and progresses proximally, affecting the whole colon. In 10% of cases the terminal ileum is also affected.

48. (a) F.
    (b) T.
    (c) F.
    (d) T.
    (e) T.

CDH is more common in girls and after malpresentation at birth. There is a familial tendency to the condition. The condition should be diagnosed by routine clinical examination of the newborn baby and subsequent follow-up examinations. Abduction of the hip tends to be restricted, and gentle manual abduction of the hip may be accompanied by a clunk (Ortolani's test) which can be felt if the examiner's fingers are placed behind the hip joint. The diagnosis can be confirmed with ultrasound. X-ray examination is used far less due to the potential risk of irradiation to the gonads. Asymmetry of the groin skin creases should alert the examiner to a possible unilateral CDH.

In the majority of children, CDH that is detected will resolve with conservative treatment. Splintage with the hip flexed and abducted should be started as soon as the diagnosis is confirmed. If the joint capsule shortens in this position the prognosis is excellent. Very rarely the hip will not reduce and open reduction is then required. Undetected CDH or late presentation is associated with secondary osteoarthritis and a poor outcome.

49. (a) F.
    (b) F.
    (c) T.
    (d) T.
    (e) F.

Nipple discharge is relatively uncommon but may be very alarming to the patient. Serous, serosanguinous or bloody discharges are usually due to hyperplastic conditions – commonly duct papilloma but also hyperplasia, carcinoma *in situ*, or carcinoma; less commonly due to duct ectasia. The risk of carcinoma rises with age from under 3% at 40 to over 30% above the age of 60 years. Coloured (green/brown) discharge is usually related to duct ectasia or a cyst, whilst galactorrhoea may be physiological or due to hyperprolactinaemia. Management involves excluding important causes (mammography may be useful), and is then dependent on symptoms, but an associated lump should be treated 'on its merits' and as a priority.

50. (a) F.
    (b) F.
    (c) T.
    (d) T.
    (e) T.

Ostium secundum defects cause a left atrium to right atrium shunt which is acyanotic (as apposed to a right-to-left shunt). The shunt is usually small at birth as pulmonary arterial pressure is high but, as pulmonary pressure falls, the shunt increases and symptoms may result, but often not until late childhood or beyond. Symptoms include breathlessness on exertion, tiredness or recurrent chest infections. Often, the child will present with an asymptomatic murmur associated with fixed splitting of the second heart sound due to delayed closure of the pulmonary valve, secondary to increased pulmonary blood flow. Chest X-ray reveals a large heart and pulmonary artery with pulmonary plethora, whilst an electrocardiogram (ECG) may reveal right ventricular hypertrophy, right axis deviation and right bundle branch block. Cardiac catheterization is required to determine accurately the degree of shunting. If pulmonary blood flow is found to be twice systemic flow, then surgical closure of the defect using cardiopulmonary bypass is recommended.

Answers to Paper 3

1. (a) T.
   (b) F.
   (c) F.
   (d) T.
   (e) T.

   The risk of recurrent thromboembolism is greatest for the first few weeks after the initial event. Although the evidence is conflicting, and the risk is also dependent on the extent of the initial thrombotic episode, most patients are treated for a minimum of 3 months with anticoagulation. Warfarin is commonly used for this, but as it crosses the placenta and can cause fetal damage, heparin is used in pregnant women. This may be given subcutaneously, the dose being determined by the activated partial thromboplastin time (APTT).

   Surgical removal of an extensive iliofemoral vein thrombus is possible, but not without risk. Rethrombosis rate is high and there is no evidence that this reduces venous valve damage or prevents the development of a post-phlebitic limb. Thrombectomy is usually only undertaken when the thrombus is extensive, limb swelling massive (with a risk of venous gangrene) and the history short (less than 5 days). Filters can be placed in the inferior vena cava and will prevent large emboli from reaching the lungs. They may have a role in patients with large free-floating thrombi, when recurrent pulmonary emboli have occurred despite anticoagulation and when significant thromboembolic disease has occurred and anticoagulation is contraindicated.

   Once the patient is mobile it is usual to prescribe a below-knee graduated compression stocking in an attempt to limit the effect that the thrombus has had on venous haemodynamics.

2. (a) F.
   (b) F.
   (c) T.
   (d) F.
   (e) F.
   Sudden loss of circulating blood or plasma may result in shock, when the nutritional demands of the tissues cannot be met by the reduced cardiac output. Homeostatic mechanisms act to maintain blood pressure initially, so the pulse rises and urine output falls to below normal levels of 1 ml/kg per hour. Respiratory rate may rise to enhance blood oxygenation and peripheral vasoconstriction occurs to maintain blood pressure and thus cerebral perfusion. Central venous pressure (CVP) measurements are useful to monitor responses to treatment but a single reading is of limited value as CVP reflects right ventricular function, not left. (Although in a normal, healthy heart they are, obviously, matched.) Pulmonary artery wedge pressure measurement via a Swan–Ganz catheter may be of more use and also allows the estimation of cardiac output by thermodilution.

3. (a) F.
   (b) T.
   (c) F.
   (d) T.
   (e) F.
   Grave's disease is an autoimmune condition where the IgG thyroid stimulating immunoglobulin (TSI) results in hyperthyroidism and a vascular goitre, over which may be heard a bruit. It may be treated with antithyroid drugs, but recurrence is common; with radio-iodine, after which hypothyroidism is common; or subtotal thyroidectomy. Surgery is safe provided that cardiovascular manifestations of thyrotoxicosis have been controlled by beta blockers, or the patient is first rendered euthyroid pharmacologically.

4. (a) F.
   (b) F.

(c) F.
(d) T.
(e) T.
A ganglion is a localized, tense, firm, cystic swelling containing clear, gelatinous fluid. The cause is uncertain but they invariably occur adjacent to a tendon sheath or joint capsule so they may result from a leakage of synovial fluid. They are most commonly seen on the dorsum of the wrist or foot. They may be painful and usually appear firm to touch. The traditional remedy used to be hitting them with the family Bible or other heavy object, but this technique is painful and is associated with a high recurrence rate. Some claim good results by aspiration and steroid injection, but this is technically difficult (the fluid is very viscous) and has not become popular. The usual treatment is careful, complete surgical excision (augmented by the use of a tourniquet to produce a bloodless field), but there is a significant recurrence rate.

5. (a) T.
   (b) F.
   (c) T.
   (d) T.
   (e) T.
Aortic valve replacement may be indicated for aortic valve regurgitation or stenosis when severe or associated with complications such as angina or left ventricular hypertrophy. The operation is performed via a median sternotomy and cardiopulmonary bypass is required whilst the aorta is clamped to perform the replacement. Usually a prosthetic valve is inserted. This requires long-term oral anticoagulant therapy to reduce the risk of thrombus forming on the valve, whilst systemic antibiotics are required during procedures that produce bacteraemia (such as dental extraction) to prevent graft infection.
Occasionally, a heterograft (rendered non-immunogenic by tanning with gluteraldehyde) is used. This reduces the need for anticoagulation and may be indicated in elderly, frail patients, but the long-term valve performance is inferior to prosthetic valves.

6. (a) T.
   (b) F.
   (c) T.
   (d) F.
   (e) F.

   The peak incidence of Crohn's disease is in the age range 20–40 years affecting 5 in 100 000 of the population (more commonly in men than in women). The inflammatory process is transmural, explaining the high incidence (30%) of fistulas. A number of systemic manifestations may occur, including EN, sclerosing cholangitis, finger clubbing and aphthous mouth ulcers. The principle of surgery is to deal with the complications of the disease. Removal of involved bowel found at operation does not prevent further complications. Many patients require multiple operations with removal of segments of badly diseased bowel, and may develop the short bowel syndrome, so bowel should be preserved when possible. It is sometimes possible to relieve an obstruction by performing a 'stricturoplasty', so preserving bowel length. Crohn's colitis may require total colectomy, but the terminal ileum may develop Crohn's and so ileoanal pouch construction is not undertaken.

7. (a) F.
   (b) T.
   (c) T.
   (d) T.
   (e) F.

   Most lumbar disc prolapses occur in the lower lumbar spine at L4/5 or L5/S1, and 10% involve both levels. Disc protrusion is usually posterolateral, producing local pain or root signs such as reduced ankle jerks and pain down the back of the thigh and lateral aspect of the leg with L5/S1 prolapse. However, 2% of discs prolapse centrally and may result in bilateral sciatic root irritation or sphincter paralysis. Although often preceded by a long history of lower back ache, the acute episode is often precipitated by bending or lifting, especially if rotation occurs at the same time. In most cases treatment is bed-rest, analgesia, traction and, occasionally, manipulation. Repeated attacks, progressive neurological deficit and central prolapse are indications for surgical intervention.

8. (a) F.
   (b) T.
   (c) F.
   (d) T.
   (e) F.

Hypospadias is a common congenital condition affecting 1 in 300–500 boys. The distal urethra fails to develop and the meatus opens on the urethral surface of the penis (to a varying degree – very slightly off-centre, down the penile shaft or even perineal). The distal urethra is replaced by a contracted fibrous band which causes ventral flexion of the penis (chordee). The characteristic deformity is completed by a hooded foreskin, which is deficient ventrally. Mild deformity requires no treatment, but more severe cases need surgical correction, usually in two stages. The first operation is to straighten the chordee deformity and the second brings the meatus to the tip of the penis, usually by constructing a tube from the foreskin. Circumcision is thus contraindicated in boys with hypospadias.

9. (a) T.
   (b) T.
   (c) F.
   (d) F.
   (e) T.

Obstruction of the biliary tree by gallstones or tumour causes dilatation of the bile ducts that is seen on ultrasound scanning. Bilirubin is conjugated in the liver but cannot pass into the small bowel and so conjugated bilirubinaemia and then bilirubinuria results, producing dark urine. The bowel becomes devoid of bile salts and so urobilinogen cannot be formed, stools become pale; and vitamin K is not absorbed resulting in a deficiency of vitamin K-dependent clotting factors II, VII, IX and X.

10. (a) F.
    (b) T.

(c) F.
(d) F.
(e) T.

Insertion of an intercostal tube drain may be required for drainage of air (pneumothorax), fluid (pleural effusion), blood (haemothorax), pus (empyema) or prophylactically following thoracic surgery. The side of insertion should be confirmed clinically and radiologically. For pneumothorax, the second intercostal space, midclavicular line, is a convenient but cosmetically poor location; the 4th/5th space, midaxillary line is a better alternative. A basal drain is used to drain fluid. Under local anaesthesia, the tissues should be separated by blunt dissection, through the intercostal space to the pleura. The drain should then slip in with minimal force, as any firm pressure is obviously dangerous. Intercostal vessels run just under a rib and should ideally be avoided, but it is a mistake to use a small drain as drainage may not be adequate. Connection to an underwater seal system ensures a one-way passage of air.

11. (a) F.
    (b) F.
    (c) T.
    (d) T.
    (e) T.

Vomiting causes loss of H^+ ions, resulting in alkalosis. The kidney compensates by preserving Na^+ and H^+ and thus excretes K^+, causing hypokalaemia. Eventually, this mechanism is overcome and the kidney also excretes H^+ in order to preserve sodium, resulting in 'paradoxical aciduria'. Alkalosis causes the lungs to retain CO_2 to compensate, and in severe cases leads to prolonged periods of apnoea and Cheyne–Stoke's respiration. A severe alkalosis and dehydration may induce renal epithelial damage and failure.

12. (a) F.
    (b) F.
    (c) T.

(d) T.
(e) F.

Clinical diagnosis alone is not accurate enough. The diagnosis is usually made with venography or (increasingly) with duplex ultrasound. Iodine-125 fibrinogen uptake is very sensitive, but is not used routinely as iodine uptake by the thyroid must be blocked first which takes 48 hours. Recent concern regarding HIV and blood products together with the improvements in duplex ultrasound suggest that this test will rarely, if ever, be used in the future.

Most patients are empirically kept on bed-rest with their legs elevated until fully anticoagulated. This is supposed to allow adherence of the thrombus to the vein wall, but there is no evidence for this although swelling is reduced. Fifty per cent of DVTs are silent and so reliance cannot be placed on the development of clinical signs or symptoms for their detection.

13. (a) T.
    (b) F.
    (c) F.
    (d) F.
    (e) T.

The principle of surgical treatment is to resect the tumour together with the lymphatics draining it. These run with the arteries, so for a right-sided tumour a right hemicolectomy with ligation of the right colic and ileocaecal arteries would be undertaken. If the lesion causes obstruction this needs to be relieved surgically. A proximal defunctioning stoma can be fashioned, then subsequently removed along with the tumour. Alternatively, the tumour can be resected at the first operation. If a right hemicolectomy is undertaken, primary anastomosis is usually possible. If a left colonic lesion is resected then either a proximal defunctioning colostomy can be fashioned (Hartmann's procedure) which may be closed at a subsequent operation or a primary anastomosis performed after on-table lavage of the bowel to clear faecal material. Flatus tubes may be useful in the management of pseudo-obstruction where there is no mechanical blockage.

Post-operative radiotherapy can reduce the recurrence rate of local rectal tumours, but does not improve survival. The role of pre-operative radiotherapy is being evaluated. CEA may rise after treatment which is suggestive of recurrent disease, but a high initial level does not signify spread of the primary tumour. A small group of patients have more than one tumour at presentation.

14. (a) F.
    (b) F.
    (c) T.
    (d) T.
    (e) F.

In the majority of cases no cause for the hydrocele is found. Occasionally, secondary hydroceles result from heart failure, testicular tumours, injury or infection. In adults they are not associated with hernias, although both conditions are relatively common. In an elderly man it would not be necessary to obtain an ultrasound scan of the testicle if it was normal on clinical examination after aspiration of the hydrocele fluid. Treatment is only required if the hydrocele is symptomatic. Aspiration alone is of little value as the fluid re-collects, although the instillation of a sclerosant may prevent recurrence and is advocated by some surgeons. Surgical excision can be carried out, but scrotal haematomas can occur. Plication of the sac (Lord's procedure) leaves a slightly bulky mass behind the scrotum, but is claimed to be less likely to cause a haematoma as little scrotal dissection is required.

15. (a) T.
    (b) T.
    (c) F.
    (d) F.
    (e) T.

Portal hypertension may result from pre-hepatic causes (e.g. portal vein thrombosis), hepatic causes (cirrhosis) or post-hepatic causes (hepatic vein obstruction, e.g. Budd–Chiari syndrome). It causes hypersplenism and gastrointestinal bleeding from varices (portosystemic collaterals) – typically at the gastro-oesophageal junction, but anal varices also occur. Haemorrhoids are not anal varices. Ascites commonly complicates portal hypertension due to hepatic or post-hepatic causes when liver function is compromised, but is uncommonly associated with portal vein thrombosis. Bleeding oesophageal varices are usually managed conservatively and/or by injection sclerotherapy, but in selected cases surgical decompression may be indicated.

16. (a) T.
    (b) F.
    (c) T.
    (d) T.
    (e) F.

Secretory otitis media is due to obstruction of the eustachian tubes due to enlargement of the adenoids or upper-respiratory-tract infections. Rarely, in an adult a nasopharyngeal tumour may block the tube on one side. It commonly causes deafness in children, but unless complicated is not usually painful or associated with discharge. Treatment is to remove the cause of obstruction to the eustachian tubes if possible. If it recurs then grommets are inserted in the drum.

17. (a) F.
    (b) T.
    (c) F.
    (d) T.
    (e) T.

Popliteal aneurysm, DVT, Baker's cyst, muscle tears or osteoarthritis may all cause pain behind the knee. However, it is important to identify the cause rapidly, as immediate treatment may be required. Although surgery increases the risk of DVT, it can occur after periods of immobility, secondary to illness or long-distance travel, especially if there has been a previous DVT. Popliteal aneurysms may thrombose or embolize, causing distal ischaemia. They can rarely rupture. Likewise, a Baker's cyst, which is a herniation of the synovial joint, may present as a tender swelling or, if it ruptures, as pain which may spread down the calf. Tears of the calf muscles can occur after relatively minor injury such as a missed footing on a stairway. Other swellings in the popliteal fossa, such as neuromas, can occur and so the diagnosis must be firmly established before embarking on surgical removal.

Clinically it can be very difficult to distinguish between these conditions and duplex ultrasound is becoming increasingly useful as the associated technology improves. Cystic swellings can be distinguished from popliteal aneurysms, especially if the equipment is colour-coded for flow, and calf vein DVTs can be visualized. This allows identification of conditions which may need immediate treatment.

18. (a) F.
    (b) F.
    (c) F.
    (d) F.
    (e) T.

Following a severe head injury the commonest causes of death in those who survive the initial event are obstruction of the airway or other injuries sustained. Attention must be directed to these, especially the airway. Blood loss can be massive from the head injury alone, especially if the scalp has been lacerated.

Apart from the most urgent cases, computerized tomography (CT) scanning is carried out before intervention in order to locate accurately treatable intracranial haematomas and prevent unnecessary surgery on patients with cerebral oedema alone or massive, unsalvagable brain injury. Extradural haematomas commonly occur following a fracture of the temporal bone which tears the middle meningeal artery. Extradural haematomas are less common than subdural bleeding because shearing forces tend to tear subdural vessels, especially in the elderly. Subdural bleeding commonly occurs after head injury and may cause symptoms similar to meningitis.

The importance of extradural haematomas lies in their early recognition. They may follow a relatively minor injury, sometimes associated with loss of consciousness. The patient then appears reasonably well (the lucid interval) and often a fracture is not seen or is missed on skull X-ray. The torn middle meningeal artery continues to bleed, stripping the dura off the inside of the skull and giving the haematoma its characteristic lentiform shape on CT scan. The haematoma causes increased intracranial pressure and the patient's level of consciousness decreases. The increased pressure causes herniation of the temporal lobe of the brain and stretching of the oculomotor nerve as it runs across the base of the skull. The sympathetic fibres which supply the pupil run with this nerve and stretching results in dilatation of the pupil, initially on the ipsilateral side of the haematoma, but eventually on both sides. This is a very grave sign and implies that, without immediate intervention, death will occur. The haematoma can be evacuated with a burr hole over the pterion and the bleeding vessel controlled via a limited craniectomy.

19. (a) F.
    (b) F.
    (c) T.
    (d) T.
    (e) F.

Basal cell carcinomas present as spreading ulcers (rodent ulcers) or a flat papule, usually on the upper face. They are locally destructive but very rarely metastasize. Exposure to sunlight is a pre-disposing factor and they are therefore seen in elderly fair-skinned men, especially those who have had an outdoor occupation. Rodent ulcers are effectively treated by radiotherapy (where skin grafting would be difficult or disfiguring) or surgical excision (when radiotherapy would damage underlying cartilage), depending on position and extent of spread.

20. (a) F.
    (b) T.
    (c) F.
    (d) T.
    (e) T.
    Gas gangrene results from a mixed infection with saccharolytic (e.g. *Clostridium welchii*) and proteolytic (e.g. *Clostridium sporogenes*) *Clostridia*. Contamination must be accompanied by reduced tissue oxygenation for gas gangrene to occur. Thus gangrene is most commonly seen in badly contused, lacerated war or agricultural wounds complicated by foreign-body implantation. Although gas gangrene is traditionally a complication of amputation it is now very rare, possibly due to routine antibiotic prophylaxis. Exotoxins induce muscle necrosis and gas formation. Initially the affected area becomes tense, oedematous and crepitant, later with the production of a foul odour and greenish-black appearance resulting from muscle putrefaction, associated with profound systemic disturbance with shock. Non-gas forming *Clostridia* may result in the absence of crepitus or visible gas on X-ray. Principles of treatment are resuscitation, high doses of systemic antibiotics and urgent radical surgical debridement. Hyperbaric oxygen reduces mortality and is indicated, if available.

21. (a) T.
    (b) F.
    (c) T.
    (d) F.
    (e) F.
    Known risk factors for gastric cancer include type B atrophic gastritis (associated with PA) and achlorhydria (hypoacidosis), e.g. secondary to previous partial gastrectomy. This may allow gastric colonization by bacteria which produce carcinogens such as nitrosamines. Local symptoms include dyspepsia, dysphagia or gastric outflow obstruction, but the diagnosis should be considered in a patient with iron deficiency anaemia, especially if associated with anorexia, weight loss or

cachexia. Spread is locally to adjacent structures and commonly to local lymphatics, then blood borne to the liver. Transcoelomic spread may occur to all over the peritoneal cavity, classically to the ovaries. Prognosis is related to the extent of spread at presentation, as the only hope of cure is radical surgery.

22. (a) F.
    (b) T.
    (c) F.
    (d) F.
    (e) T.

The knee joint comprises the patellofemoral and the medial and lateral tibiofemoral articulations. OA commonly affects the knee joint, especially the patellofemoral articulation followed by the medial femorotibial joint. This results in fibrillation and destruction of the articular cartilage, with formation of osteophytes and loose bodies. Synovial proliferation generally occurs with excess synovial fluid production which can be detected as an effusion. OA may be primary or secondary to previous injury or deformity. The knee joint is the commonest large joint to be affected by rheumatoid arthritis and the destruction caused may result in secondary OA.

Treatment should initially be conservative: weight reduction, anti-inflammatory and analgesic drugs and occasionally intra-articular injections of steroids. If this fails then tibial osteotomy may be very effective. The results of total knee replacement are satisfactory, but not as good as for the hip due to the mechanical instability of the knee. Arthrodesis is rarely undertaken, as a fused knee imposes severe restriction of mobility.

23. (a) T.
    (b) T.
    (c) F.
    (d) T.
    (e) F.

Strictures of the urethra may be caused by congenital abnormalities of the urethra, but more commonly follow trauma (including surgical instrumentation) or infection. The diagnosis can be made from the symptoms of reduced stream, frequency and a poor flow rate. Urethrography or urethroscopy are usually diagnostic. Treatment can be by dilatation (bouginage), incision of the stricture (urethrotomy), or urethroplasty. Excision of the stricture and end-to-end repair is not usually possible unless the stricture is very short, and often results in recurrence.

24. (a) T.
    (b) F.
    (c) F.
    (d) T.
    (e) T.

Oesophageal atresia is associated with maternal hydramnios. It may occur alone or with TOF. Various anomalies are seen but the commonest is a blind proximal oesophageal pouch, with the distal oesophagus connecting the trachea to the stomach. The baby cannot vomit but presents with cough, copious sputum, gastric dilatation and respiratory difficulties. Urgent intervention is necessary to prevent acid aspiration. This involves gastrostomy and ligation of the TOF. Primary oesophago-oesophageal anastomosis is possible in over half of cases, but cervical oesophagostomy may be necessary, with subsequent reconstruction with colonic interposition or free-jejunal transplant. TOF may be associated with the 'vacterl' syndrome – **v**ertebral, **a**nal, **c**ardiac, **t**racheo-**o**esophageal, **r**enal and **l**imb abnormalities. Mortality is 50%, but the prognosis is excellent in babies without associated abnormalities or established aspiration pneumonia.

25. (a) T.
    (b) F.
    (c) T.
    (d) F.
    (e) F.

The pre-patellar bursa lies subcutaneously anterior to the patella. Inflammation occurs if it is chronically irritated, for instance by working on bent knees as carpet layers do.

There is no association with osteoarthritis. It is not usually of bacterial origin, but organisms can enter through broken skin and, if there is marked redness, local tenderness associated with a pyrexia then infection must be suspected. Aspiration can be performed and may relieve symptoms, but more importantly may identify infection when there is suspicion. Treatment is rest, anti-inflammatory agents and analgesia. If infection is suspected, antibiotics are also given. If there is overt infection the bursa may initially need to be drained. If the condition is recurrent and the symptoms marked the bursa should be removed surgically.

26. (a) T.
    (b) F.
    (c) F.
    (d) T.
    (e) T.

Acute otitis media is an infection of the middle ear caused by bacteria entering from the nasopharynx or sometimes via a perforated drum. Treatment is analgesia and antibiotics which will cure most attacks. If this fails or there is residual pus in the middle ear incision of the drum (myringotomy) will relieve the symptoms and reduce the risk of complications including deafness or spread to the mastoid or meninges. Occasionally the drum bursts spontaneously with discharge of pus and resolution. Plastic drainage tubes (grommets) are used for recurrent secretory otitis media, not infections.

27. (a) T.
    (b) F.
    (c) F.
    (d) T.
    (e) F.

Scalds are more likely to produce superficial burns. Contact or electrical burns are often deep. Loss of sensation suggests a full-thickness burn, but is not totally reliable. Estimation of burn extent is important for prognostic reasons and to predict fluid requirements. The 'rule of nines' is used and the head and neck comprise 9%

of the total area. Children probably require hospital admission for partial-thickness burns over about 10%, for full-thickness burns over 2–5% of surface area, or if the head, hands or genitals are involved.

28. (a) F.
    (b) T.
    (c) F.
    (d) T.
    (e) F.

Antibiotic prophylaxis should be given to such a patient to reduce the risk of post-operative sepsis and wound infection. The regimen chosen should ensure that maximal tissue concentrations of an antibiotic that is effective against the expected contaminants are attained at the time of surgery. Thus intravenous antibiotics are given (locally applied agents are ineffective) perioperatively. Three doses are given traditionally, but a single per-operative dose is probably just as effective. Anaerobes (e.g. *Bacteroides*) and Gram-negative bacilli (e.g. *Escherichia coli*) are the likely pathogens following large bowel surgery, so metronidazole is usually given, combined with a broad-spectrum antibiotic active against Gram-negative organisms.

29. (a) T.
    (b) T.
    (c) T.
    (d) T.
    (e) F.

Most nasal polyps are multiple benign oedematous areas of mucous membrane associated with hypersensitivity and have no malignant potential. Solitary polyps may rarely be malignant. The polyps may cause nasal discharge, obstruction and prevent drainage of the sinuses. If large and symptomatic they should be removed surgically, but smaller polyps and areas of oedematous mucosa may respond well to steroid nasal sprays.

30. (a) T.
    (b) F.

(c) F.
(d) T.
(e) F.

In the UK, carcinoma of the stomach presents with symptoms of dyspepsia, but after spread to the lymphatics surgical cure is impossible. To achieve earlier diagnosis, all except young patients with dyspepsia need early endoscopy. Empirical H_2-receptor antagonists may mask symptoms and delay diagnosis, but after the diagnosis has been confirmed they are useful for reducing symptoms. Palliative gastrectomy is the usual treatment. Gastric cancer is not radiosensitive and trials of adjuvant chemotherapy continue. In this country, 5-year survival is closer to 5% than 50%.

31. (a) T.
(b) F.
(c) F.
(d) T.
(e) T.

Cardiac complications are the commonest cause of mortality during aortic surgery. History and clinical examination including resting ECG are not reliable, because many patients have silent myocardial ischaemia. Dipyridamole thallium scanning, echocardiography or exercise ECG are better methods of assessment, although the cost benefit in aortic surgery is not established.

Ultrasound scanning will determine that an aneurysm is infrarenal and give an accurate indication of size in the majority of cases. CT scanning may demonstrate the renal vessels in difficult cases and provides information about other structures such as the kidney and iliac arteries. Inflammatory aneurysms can be identified by a thick halo of soft tissue around the aneurysm sac and, as the surgical risks for repair of these aneurysms are greater, this might influence management. Angiography is relatively invasive and reserved for difficult cases such as the association with occlusive disease or for high aneurysms when visceral arteries may be involved. Angiography only demonstrates the lumen of the aneurysm and so gives little information about size.

Infection of aortic prostheses is uncommon but catastrophic. For this reason antibiotic prophylaxis is given on induction of anaesthesia. There is no evidence that more than one dose is necessary, but many surgeons give three doses. The commonest infecting organisms are *Staphylococci* and the regimen used should cover these at least. The parasympathetic plexus around the lower aorta is involved with penile erection and, if this is damaged during aortic surgery, impotence may result. The patient should be warned of this prior to surgery.

32. (a) F.
    (b) F.
    (c) T.
    (d) F.
    (e) F.

Day-case surgery is becoming popular as it is cost-effective and avoids overnight hospital stays and is therefore popular with patients. Its increase has arisen from a change in thinking rather than new technological innovation. Day surgery requires a dedicated unit, experienced staff and careful patient selection. The decision as to the suitability of day surgery is based on the type of operation, the fitness of the patient and the social circumstances of the patient, for instance they must have someone at home with them in the early post-operative period and access to a telephone for emergencies. Many operations under general anaesthetic may now be performed as day cases, but obviously patients should not drive themselves home afterwards! Children tend to recover quickly from surgery and anaesthesia, dislike hospitals and are therefore ideal for day surgery for a large number of procedures.

33. (a) F.
    (b) T.
    (c) F.
    (d) F.
    (e) F.

Acute retention is painful and it is often reasonable to give the patient analgesia, but relief of the obstruction is the best method of pain relief. Although retention is most often caused by bladder outlet obstruction due to prostatic hypertrophy, the acute episode may be precipitated by other factors such as antidepressant drugs, pain from other sources or constipation. Sometimes correction of these problems after relief of the acute situation by passage of a catheter, may allow the patient to pass urine again without the need for surgery. Failure to pass a urethral catheter may be due to inexperience but, if not, a suprapubic catheter can be used. Some surgeons advocate the use of suprapubic catheters in the first instance to avoid damage to the urethra. Open prostatectomy is usually undertaken for very large glands when transurethral resection would take a prolonged time, but TURP is most often undertaken. The longer a catheter is left *in situ* the greater the chance of bacterial contamination of the urine. Ideally, the patient should be offered elective surgery on the next routine operating list after admission. In practice this is not always possible and the catheter has to remain for longer.

34. (a) T.
    (b) T.
    (c) T.
    (d) T.
    (e) F.

So-called 'tennis elbow' is characterized by pain over the origin of the wrist extensors on the lateral epicondyle which results in tenderness there, pain on extension of the fingers or active wrist dorsiflexion. It may follow minor repetitive injury to the extensor origin, chondromalacia of the radial head or entrapment of the radial nerve as it passes over the lateral aspect of the elbow. Treatment includes rest (if necessary, with a splint), local injections of hydrocortisone, physiotherapy and manipulation. If this fails and symptoms are severe, release of the extensor origin may relieve the symptoms.

35. (a) T.
    (b) F.
    (c) T.
    (d) T.
    (e) F.

Chronic retention is commonly due to benign prostatic hypertrophy and is not associated with bladder tumours. As the onset is gradual, discomfort may be felt but the patient is not in pain. The upper renal tracts may also become dilated and renal failure results. Relief of the obstruction may result in a diuresis due to the high urea level which acts as a diuretic, and care has to be taken to keep up with this fluid loss. If the urine is infected, antibiotics should be started and a catheter passed.

36. (a) T.
    (b) F.
    (c) F.
    (d) T.
    (e) T.

The cause of pyloric stenosis is unknown but it commonly presents in boys 4–6 weeks of age with projectile vomiting and 'failure to thrive'. The diagnosis can usually be confirmed clinically during a 'test feed', but occasionally ultrasound or barium meal may be helpful. Due to the vomiting the child is likely to have a severe hypochlorhydric metabolic alkalosis and so, once the diagnosis has been confirmed, time (usually 24–36 hours) is needed to resuscitate the baby. This includes nasogastric suction and intravenous saline until the serum chloride concentration climbs above 100 mmol/l. Definitive treatment is by pyloromyotomy (Ramstedt's operation), under general anaesthetic with every attempt to keep the child warm, the thickened muscles of the pylorus are split, allowing the mucosa to bulge free. Oral fluids can usually be recommenced 4 hours after surgery.

37. (a) T.
    (b) F.
    (c) T.

(d) T.
(e) T.
Acute aortic dissection involves haemorrhagic intramural separation of the aortic media, often caused by cystic medial necrosis. The resulting 'false' passage may occlude the origin of any of the aortic branches. Thus dissection presents with chest pain and collapse, followed by death; or any combination of stroke, upper or lower limb ischaemia, paraplegia, renal failure or gut ischaemia. Dissection is most commonly seen in middle-aged male hypertensives. Clinical diagnosis is confirmed by aortography, computerized tomography (CT) scanning or echocardiography. Dissection of the ascending aorta may spread back to the aortic valve and cause incompetence, coronary artery occlusion or pericardial tamponade. Initial treatment is urgently to control high blood pressure. Ascending aortic dissections (type A) should then be treated by replacement of the aortic valve and ascending aorta. Stable descending aortic lesions may be treated medically by long-term antihypertensive drugs, but signs of major vessel occlusion (e.g. anuria, and acute leg ischaemia) require surgical intervention.

38. (a) T.
    (b) F.
    (c) F.
    (d) T.
    (e) T.
Acute cholecystitis usually results from a gallstone impacting in the cystic duct, causing gallbladder distension and secondary infection (but acalculous cholecystitis may occasionally complicate severe systemic illness). The patient is unwell, pyrexial and tender in the right upper quadrant of the abdomen. There is usually a neutrophil leucocytosis, and serum transaminases and amylase may be moderately raised. The diagnosis is confirmed by ultrasound and the treatment is by resuscitation and usually early cholecystectomy. Fatty food intolerance was once thought to be a chronic symptom of gallstones, but is now known to be as frequent in people without gallstones.

39. (a) F.
    (b) F.
    (c) T.
    (d) T.
    (e) T.

Up to 10% of the population may suffer Raynaud's phenomenon, but in the majority of cases the symptoms are mild and there is no identifiable associated condition (primary Raynaud's phenomenon). The diagnosis is based on the history and clinical signs (if any), but abnormal rewarming patterns after making the hand cold can be seen with thermography and may confirm the diagnosis.

Treatment consists of avoidance of and protection against cold exposure. Some drugs such as nifedipine and intravenous prostacyclin have been claimed to be beneficial, but long-term results are usually poor. If severe, digital ulceration and gangrene occur and obliteration of digital vessels on angiography can be seen. Sympathectomy may help to overcome the exacerbation.

In a small number of patients there will be an associated condition (secondary Raynaud's phenomenon) such as rheumatoid arthritis, systemic lupus erythematosus or, rarely, a malignancy. Cervical ribs are claimed to occasionally cause secondary Raynaud's phenomenon, and exposure to vibrating machinery is associated with a related vasospastic condition, vibration white finger. Treatment of the underlying condition is undertaken, but the outlook for patients with secondary Raynaud's phenomenon is generally less good.

40. (a) F.
    (b) F.
    (c) F.
    (d) F.
    (e) T.

A small bowel fistula is most likely to result from trauma, Crohn's disease or a complication of abdominal surgery. Output from a proximal small bowel fistula is likely to be high and result in malnutrition and fluid and electrolyte depletion. Skin excoriation and digestion of the abdominal wall is also in danger. Treatment, therefore, involves intravenous fluids and parenteral nutrition with reduced oral intake, together with adequate sump suction of the fistula with skin protection. Associated abscesses require drainage. Most fistulas heal, provided there is no distal obstruction.

41. (a) F.
    (b) T.
    (c) T.
    (d) T.
    (e) F.

The sympathetic nerve supply to the upper limbs arises from the upper thoracic sympathetic ganglia (2–5) which run along the upper thorax on the necks of the ribs. In the neck, the sympathetic ganglia fuse to form three large ganglia. The lower cervical ganglion is usually fused with the T1 ganglia to form the stellate ganglion and damage to this results in constriction of the pupil, ptosis and absence of sweating on the ipsilateral side of the face (Horner's syndrome).

Surgical destruction or removal of the T2 ganglia (especially for conditions of the hand) and T3 and T4 ganglia (it is difficult to reach T5 and not usually necessary) can give good results for severe hyperhydrosis of the hand. The initial results for Raynaud's phenomenon are variable and the long-term results poor. It is useful for exacerbations of the condition, especially if there is digital ulceration or gangrene and when other treatments have failed. Other conditions in which sympathectomy may be used include causalgia and severe ischaemia (combined with revascularization procedures), although evidence of benefit is largely anecdotal in these situations.

The procedure may be carried out by a superclavicular route (hence cervical sympathectomy) or by a transthoracic route (usually through the 3/4 interspace in the axilla). These are quite major procedures and the use of the thoracoscope allows upper thoracic sympathectomy to be performed with less risk.

42. (a) T.
    (b) F.
    (c) T.
    (d) T.
    (e) F.
    Blood is stored at 4°C and so red blood cells lose their 2,3-diphosphoglycerate activity which impairs their ability to release oxygen. Blood stored in citrate risks lowered ionized calcium levels, whilst increased pH and potassium levels may impair myocardial function. Platelet and leucocyte aggregates may be responsible for ARDS. Stored blood has few functioning platelets and is deficient in clotting factors, pre-disposing to coagulopathies.

43. (a) T.
    (b) F.
    (c) F.
    (d) T.
    (e) T.
    Phaeochromocytoma is a rare tumour arising from sympathetic nervous tissue and presents with a host of possible symptoms related to excessive catecholamine production, usually hypertension: 10% are malignant, 10% arise from a site other than an adrenal gland and 10% are bilateral. It may be associated with the familial MEN II syndrome with medullary cell carcinoma of the thyroid and parathyroid adenoma. Localized urinary excretion of catecholamine metabolites is seen and even smaller tumours are localized effectively by CT scanning. Treatment is surgical excision with careful per-operative blood pressure control with α- and β-adrenocepter blockade.

44. (a) F.
    (b) T.
    (c) F.
    (d) T.
    (e) F.
    Sebaceous (keratinous) cysts occur due to obstruction of the duct of a pilosebaceous follicle. The retention cyst fills with fat, epithelial cells and keratin to form a foetid, putty-

like substance and the punctum of the duct may be seen at the summit of the cyst. They are usually adherent to the skin. Cysts usually occur in areas where there are many sebaceous ducts – the face and scalp in particular, where they are often multiple. They do not occur on the palms of the hands or soles of the feet which are devoid of hair and, therefore, of pilosebaceous follicles. Cysts may become infected. Elective surgery involves excising the cyst. The wall of the cyst *must* be fully removed or recurrence is likely.

45. (a) F.
    (b) T.
    (c) T.
    (d) T.
    (e) F.

Deep wounds to the wrist should be formally explored to remove foreign material and identified unsuspected damage such as nerve injuries. Preliminary X-rays may identify radio-opaque foreign material, including some glass, and also detect bone damage. This should be carried out by an experienced surgeon using a tourniquet to enable good visualization. General anaesthesia can be used, but regional blocks such as axillary or brachial plexus blocks are entirely satisfactory. Biers' block, providing it is carried out by a clinician experienced with the technique and who will be in attendance throughout the procedure, is also acceptable.

Providing there is no gross contamination of the wound, results of primary tendon repair are better than subsequent repair. Nerve injuries should also be repaired using microsurgery techniques.

46. (a) T.
    (b) T.
    (c) F.
    (d) F.
    (e) T.

Hoarseness is the commonest presentation, but in advanced case laryngeal tumours may present as stridor. Malignant tumours commonly arise on the true cord, but tend to present earlier due to voice changes than those in the supra and subglottic region. Benign tumours such as nodules, polyps and papillomas are relatively uncommon and can be removed endoscopically. Hyperkeratosis is found on the true cords and occasionally may undergo malignant change.

47. (a) T.
    (b) T.
    (c) F.
    (d) F.
    (e) F.

Splenectomy is indicated electively for some haematological conditions, including hereditary spherocytosis and idiopathic thrombocytopaenic purpura, or urgently following trauma. Many patients develop a transient thrombocytosis. A subphrenic abscess may occur due to infection of a haematoma in the splenic bed or operative damage to the stomach or pancreas. There is an increased risk of overwhelming sepsis following splenectomy, especially in children. *Pneumococcus* is the commonest pathogen but the risk of *Haemophilus influenzae, Neisseria meningitidis* and *Escherichia coli* is also increased. Multivalent pneumococcal vaccine is effective in reducing the risk, but ideally needs to be given before splenectomy as the spleen is involved in affecting immunity. Following emergency splenectomy, the vaccine should be given as soon as possible post-operatively. Children should be given continuous antibiotic prophylaxis following splenectomy. This is controversial in adults. The risk of overwhelming sepsis is small, but still 10 times that of non-splenectomized individuals.

48. (a) T.
    (b) F.
    (c) F.
    (d) F.
    (e) T.

A careful history should be taken, but the important decision as to whether to perform laparotomy is mainly based on physical examination. Involuntary guarding of abdominal muscles and rebound tenderness suggests peritonitis, but both have subtle changes and findings may be difficult to interpret, especially by the inexperienced. The manoeuvre described in (d) will result in 'rebound tenderness' in most normal people! The doctor should watch the patient's face for signs of discomfort whilst finger pressure and gentle release are performed. Better still, ask the patient to cough and observe the reaction. A chest X-ray may reveal free gas under the diaphragm if a viscus is perforated. Amylase is a useful investigation in most patients as pancreatitis may mimic perforation and/or peritonitis and a positive result might save a harmful laparotomy. A high white-cell count may help to confirm clinical suspicion of acute appendicitis, but such a high figure suggests an abscess, or necrotic bowel or mesenteric ischaemia.

49. (a) T.
    (b) F.
    (c) T.
    (d) T.
    (e) F.

Rheumatoid arthritis commonly affects the hands, especially the metacarpal phalangeal joints and proximal interphalangeal joints, causing swelling and pain. Further joint destruction results in ulnar deviation of the fingers associated with swan neck and boutonniere deformities. Inflammation of the tendons and tendon sheaths may occur and can result in rupture of the tendon, especially the extensors causing a 'dropped finger'. Splintage of affected joints may produce useful reduction in pain during periods of active inflammation and also help reduce subsequent deformity. Rheumatoid factors will be undetectable in up to 20% of patients, especially early in the disease.

50. (a) F.
    (b) F.
    (c) F.

(d) T.
(e) F.
Upper-respiratory-tract infection in children may be complicated by inflammation of mesenteric lymph nodes, which may produce symptoms and signs similar to acute appendicitis. Mesenteric adenitis presents with abdominal pain associated with pharyngitis. Headache is not unusual, temperature is often raised above 38°C and cervical adenitis may co-exist. Guarding may be present, but rebound tenderness suggests appendicitis. Any doubt after a brief period of observation and surgical exploration is the safest course.

Answers to Paper 4

1. (a) F.
   (b) F.
   (c) T.
   (d) T.
   (e) F.

   The aim of surgery is usually to obtain local control rather than cure, and wide local excision of the tumour combined with radiotherapy may achieve this in many cases without the need for formal mastectomy. Involved axillary lymph nodes require surgical excision *or* radiotherapy, but the combination is associated with high morbidity, including lymphoedema of the arm. There is now very strong evidence supporting the use of tamoxifen in all post-menopausal women with breast cancer, but the role of chemotherapy in this group remains unclear.

2. (a) F.
   (b) T.
   (c) T.
   (d) T.
   (e) T.

   Acute prostatitis may be bacterial or viral, but it is often not possible to identify an organism. If suspected, treatment with antibiotics is usually prolonged as antibiotic penetration of the prostate is poor, although some antibiotics such as ciprofloxacin achieve good levels. Prostatitis may be associated with urethral instrumentation, infected residual urine due to prostatic hypertrophy or systemic infections from other sources, but it is not sexually transmitted. It may not resolve and the patient develops chronic prostatitis. An abscess may form which, if neglected, can drain into the rectum; usually it is drained surgically via the urethra using a resectoscope.

3. (a) F.
   (b) T.
   (c) F.
   (d) T.
   (e) T.

   Dupuyten's contracture is a fibrous contracture of the palmar aponeurosis. Most commonly affecting the ring finger followed by the little finger, it can extend from the base of the fingers to the wrist causing marked fixed flexion deformity of the fingers at the metacarpal-phalangeal (MCPJ) and proximal interphalangeal joints (PIPJ). The aetiology is unknown, but is said to have an autosomally dominant inheritance and to be associated with cirrhosis, diabetes and phenytoin treatment. As might be expected, most patients appear to have none of these associations. The condition is often bilateral.

   If the deformity interferes with function, usually when flexion of the MCPJ is greater than 30°, excision of the fibrous tissue will be of benefit. This may require split skin grafting to cover defects in the palmar skin. If the condition is advanced, long-standing and particularly if marked flexion is present in the PIPJ, the only solution may be amputation of the digit if it interferes with function. Steroid injections are painful and have little role to play but, rarely, if an isolated placque is painful they may cause temporary reduction of pain.

4. (a) T.
   (b) T.
   (c) F.
   (d) T.
   (e) F.

   Testicular teratomas are tumours of germ cell origin commonly affecting young men. The incidence is increasing. They present as a swollen testicle and spread early via lymphatics to the para-aortic lymph nodes, then to supradiaphragmatic nodes and lung. Serum tumour markers are often raised and serve as useful markers of treatment response. Treatment is by orchidectomy followed by radio- and chemotherapy according to stage.

Modern chemotherapy is very effective and prognosis is often excellent.

5. (a) F.
   (b) T.
   (c) F.
   (d) F.
   (e) T.

Abdominal adhesions probably occur to a certain extent after all intraperitoneal surgery as a result of trauma, ischaemia or infection of the peritoneum, which impairs fibrinolysis and allows peritoneal injury to heal with fibrinous adhesions, which may progress to fibrous adhesions. Glove powder is no longer starch and is only one cause of adhesions and should be eliminated with the introduction of powder-free gloves. Only 5% of patients who have undergone a laparotomy ever present with intestinal obstruction. Adhesion formation may be reduced by careful, aseptic, atraumatic surgery, possibly combined with a peritoneal washout. Povidine iodine, tetracycline and recombitant tissue plasminogen activator have all been claimed to reduce adhesion formation, but intravenous antibiotics are not effective.

6. (a) F.
   (b) T.
   (c) F.
   (d) F.
   (e) F.

Major burn injury results in massive loss of fluid from the burn surface, which is maximum in the first 8 hours and requires aggressive intravenous fluid replacement. Paralytic ileus is likely to preclude large volumes of oral fluid. Full-thickness burns cause sequestration and damage to red blood cells, so blood transfusion is often needed. The patient is catabolic and is likely to remain in negative nitrogen balance until skin cover is achieved. The systemic immune response is altered by burn injury and the large open areas combine to increase the risk infection.

7. (a) F.
   (b) T.
   (c) T.
   (d) F.
   (e) T.

   Stridor indicates a degree of respiratory obstruction. It may occur in asthma, but this should be identified from the history. The sudden onset in a previously fit child suggests foreign body, acute upper-respiratory-tract infection or less commonly a laryngeal tumour such as a papilloma. Unless the respiratory obstruction is very severe, a careful history, examination and chest X-ray to check for inhaled foreign bodies should be obtained. If the stridor alters with changes in position this suggests a foreign body. If airway obstruction is severe then endotracheal intubation by an experienced paediatric anaesthetist may be required. However, this should be carried out in the presence of an experienced surgeon so that if intubation is not successful tracheostomy can be undertaken immediately.

8. (a) T.
   (b) F.
   (c) T.
   (d) T.
   (e) T.

   The thoracic outlet is bounded by the clavicle, the scalenus medius muscle and the first rib. The scalenus anterior muscle divides it into a posterior compartment through which pass the roots of the brachial plexus and subclavian artery. The subclavian vein passes through the anterior compartment. Abnormalities of any of the structures forming the thoracic outlet may interfere with the neurovascular structures and produce symptoms, the thoracic outlet syndrome (TOS). A cervical rib can cause this but congenital or post-traumatic abnormalities of the first rib or clavicle can also produce TOS.

   Pain and parathesia in the upper limb are the commonest symptoms, but compression of the subclavian artery can produce symptoms of chronic ischaemia, particularly when working with the arms above the head, or an aneurysm which can thrombose or cause emboli. Venous compression is less common, but may precipitate thrombosis of the subclavian vein.

Diagnosis is difficult. Clinical signs include pain on traction, loss of radial pulse on abduction and external rotation of the arm and a bruit in the supraclavicular fossa, but these are not diagnostic. Likewise, angiography, venography and nerve conduction studies may show abnormalities, but are often normal. The options for treatment include physiotherapy, resection of the first rib (either transaxillary or supraclavicular approach), resection of a cervical rib if present or resection of the scalene muscles. The results of treatment of TOS are very variable.

9. (a) F.
   (b) T.
   (c) T.
   (d) F.
   (e) T.

Some degree of prostatic hypertrophy is almost universal in elderly men. The effect that this has on bladder function has no relationship to the size of the gland. At first the bladder hypertrophies, causing frequency and urgency. As the condition progresses though, the bladder is unable to empty fully and the residual urine may become infected. The bladder may also leak when intra-abdominal pressure increases (overflow incontinence). This may result in damage to the upper renal tracts due to back-pressure and ascending infection resulting in renal failure. Stilboestrol has no role in the treatment of benign prostatic hypertrophy.

10. (a) F.
    (b) T.
    (c) T.
    (d) T.
    (e) F.

Scaphoid fractures are common in adults after a fall on a dorsiflexed hand. Diagnosis can be difficult, but pain, tenderness or swelling in the anatomical snuff box with reduction of wrist movements after an injury should be considered diagnostic until proved otherwise. The fracture may not show on X-ray at first because of the thin cortex of the bone, but may become clear 2 weeks later. However, if there is clinical suspicion of a fracture without X-ray confirmation, the patient should be put into the appropriate plaster, which includes the thumb. This is removed before further X-ray and clinical examination 14 days later.

The most significant complication of a fractured scaphoid is avascular necrosis of the proximal part of the bone. The blood supply of the scaphoid enters at the distal pole, so fractures will tend to disrupt the nutrition of the proximal bone. This can occur following correct treatment, but is more likely if the fracture has not been immobilized when first seen and hence has serious medico-legal implications. Secondary osteoarthritis can develop, especially if avascular necrosis occurred.

Treatment is nearly always non-surgical in the first instance, but internal fixation may be attempted if there is delayed non-union.

11. (a) F.
    (b) F.
    (c) T.
    (d) T.
    (e) F.

Nosebleeding commonly arises from the anterior part of the nasal septum (Little's area) and so gentle compression of the nose will often stop the bleeding. If this is not sufficient, packing the nose may help, but packing the post-nasal space is only undertaken if these measures fail and an ENT surgeon should be involved. Most nosebleeds arise due to local problems such as burst vessel, infection, irritation or trauma. Occasionally, there may be an underlying systemic disorder such as hypertension or a coagulopathy, and these must be suspected if the bleeding is profuse, repeated and no local cause is evident. The patient should be nursed sitting up, unless hypotensive.

Reassurance is important, but sedation is generally not a good idea as it may suppress the gag reflex and the patient may aspirate blood. Nursing the patient with the head in dependency increases venous engorgement and will increase bleeding.

12. (a) F.
    (b) F.
    (c) F.
    (d) T.
    (e) F.

Portwine stains are composed of ectatic blood vessels just below the epidermis. They are present at birth and usually become more marked with age. Excision is not usually acceptable due to the scarring left. Laser therapy (pulse dye laser) has recently been used with promising results, but is still under evaluation in a few specialist centres.

13. (a) T.
    (b) F.
    (c) F.
    (d) T.
    (e) F.

Peripheral nerves may be injured by compression which usually results in contusion (neurapraxia), complete transection (neurotmesis) such as stabbing injury or disruption of the axons within an intact myelin sheath (axontmesis). PN injuries are lower motor neurone injuries, so muscle tone is reduced.

The common peroneal nerve is frequently injured as it winds around the neck of the fibula either by compression (e.g. a plaster cast) or following a fracture of the fibula. Motor function is predominantly foot dorsiflexion which is lost. Sensory loss is variable over the anterolateral aspect of the foot.

The radial nerve is prone to injury in the axilla due to pressure, e.g. crutch, as it crosses over the posterior aspect of the shaft of the humerus and at the level of the elbow associated with dislocation and fractures. Compression of the arm by tourniquet may result in damage to the nerve with wrist drop. Triceps function is usually preserved at this level.

The ulnar nerve is at risk of injury at the elbow where it may be compressed by bony deformities or fractures. At the wrist it may be involved in lacerations. This results in clawing of the little and ring finger and wasting of the intrinsic muscles of the hand. Sensation is lost over the little and ulnar side of the ring finger. In lesions above the elbow the clawing of the fingers is absent due to paralysis of the ulnar half of flexor digitorum profundus.

14. (a) T.
    (b) F.
    (c) F.
    (d) T.
    (e) F.

A pharyngeal pouch (or diverticulum) is a protrusion between the thyropharyngeus and cricopharyngeus muscles of the pharynx. It invariably occurs in an area of weakness between these two muscles, in the midline posteriorally (Killian's dehiscence). The cause is uncertain, but it is probably due to a failure of the cricopharyngeus to relax on swallowing and/or cricopharyngeus spasm, leading to increased pharyngeal pressure. The commonest presenting feature is dysphagia, then regurgitation (the pouch fills with food), gurgling, cough, aspiration, pneumonia and weight loss, usually in elderly men. The diagnosis is confirmed by barium swallow. Fibre-optic examination is difficult and risks perforation of the pouch, especially if the diagnosis is not suspected. Treatment is controversial, but most commonly the pouch is excised and a cricopharyngeus myotomy performed.

15. (a) T.
    (b) T.
    (c) T.
    (d) T.
    (e) F.

Failure of a fracture to unite may be due to infection (more common after compound fractures) or poor nutritional blood supply (worse in some bones like the tibia and in the elderly). The bone ends may be kept apart by over traction, poorly applied internal fixation or interposing soft tissue. The patient may have underlying systemic disease or the fracture may be pathological. Diagnosis can be suggested from the X-ray by failure of callus formation. Movement at the fracture site on clinical examination confirms the diagnosis. Correction of any underlying disease or deficiency and correction of any inappropriate treatment is important and may allow union. If this fails then internal fixation and bone grafting may be successful.

16. (a) F.
    (b) F.
    (c) T.
    (d) F.
    (e) T.
    Incontinence following childbirth is relatively common. Due to damage to the pelvic floor musculature the posterior wall of the bladder may prolapse after childbirth, particularly if labour was prolonged and delivery vaginal. The external sphincter of the bladder then lies outside the levator ani and the angle between the bladder and the urethra is obliterated. Increased intra-abdominal pressure causes incontinence (stress incontinence). If mild, pelvic floor exercises may improve the situation, but often a surgical procedure to repair the pelvic floor and restore the angle of the bladder neck is required. Alpha blockers reduce the external sphincter tone and make the problem worse. Infection may cause incontinence due to urgency, but not stress.

17. (a) T.
    (b) F.
    (c) F.
    (d) T.
    (e) F.
    Intussusception is the telescoping of a segment of intestine into another one. In adults it often occurs secondary to a

polyp or tumour (lead point) but in children is usually 'idiopathic', although the likely primary cause is enlarged lymph nodes due to a viral infection. Idiopathic ileocaecal intussusception presents in infants with pain, pallor, vomiting and sometimes blood-stained mucous stools (redcurrant jelly). On examination, a sausage-shaped mass is palpated in the right upper abdomen in over 50% of cases. X-rays show distended small bowel and absence of gas in the caecum. A barium enema is diagnostic and, with the addition of hydrostatic pressure, may effectively reduce the intussusception. Recurrence after such treatment is less than 5%. Failure of hydrostatic reduction, or clinical suspicion of bowel strangulation requires laparotomy and resection of the necrotic bowel.

18. (a) F.
    (b) F.
    (c) T.
    (d) T.
    (e) F.

Axillary node status is the most powerful predictor of outcome following surgery for breast cancer, but clinical examination is unreliable. Surgical sampling of the axilla is therefore becoming routine practice in many centres. Young women with positive nodes probably require adjuvant chemotherapy or oophorectomy. Post-menopausal women with axillary node involvement require tamoxifen (although there is increasing evidence that those with normal nodes may also benefit). Long-term survival is not greatly affected by the aggressiveness of local treatment, although local recurrence rates may be. Axillary clearance followed by radiotherapy gives an unacceptable incidence of lymphoedema. Wide local excision (segmental mastectomy) gives the same disease-free survival rate as mastectomy or segmental mastectomy and radiotherapy, but the local recurrence rate is higher.

19. (a) F.
    (b) T.
    (c) T.

(d) T.
(e) T.
Pre-disposing factors to the formation of calcium bilirubinate stones are biliary infections and conditions increasing the concentration of unconjugated bilirubin in bile, such as liver cirrhosis or haemolytic anaemia. Cholesterol is found in bile as molecular complexes with bile salts and phospholipids. Should bile become saturated with cholesterol (due to increased cholesterol or reduced bile salts or phospholipids) then cholesterol crystallization and stone formation will result. Conditions pre-disposing to these events include oral contraceptives, diabetes, ileal disease or resection, pregnancy and obesity. Hyperparathyroidism pre-disposes to kidney stones.

20. (a) F.
    (b) T.
    (c) T.
    (d) F.
    (e) T.

There is considerable variation in the morphology of cervical ribs. Originating from the transverse process of C7 they may be complete ossified structures articulating with the first rib or merely fibrous bands which are not apparent on X-ray. Most ribs are asymptomatic and less than 10% cause problems. Most commonly patients complain of symptoms in the hand or arm due to traction on the brachial plexus as it is stretched over the cervical rib. Much less commonly the artery can be involved, either occluded with the arm in certain positions or by the formation of a post-stenotic aneurysm which may contain thrombus which can embolize. The subclavian vein, because it lies anteriorly is not usually involved unless there is an abnormality of the first rib as well.

21. (a) F.
    (b) T.
    (c) F.
    (d) T.
    (e) F.

Healing by first intention involves epithelialization (which occurs within 2 days) and connective tissue formation (scar tissue). The latter involves fibroblasts laying down collagen and is then followed by a period of maturation. Contraction is only required in open wounds that heal by second intention. A wound never reaches the strength of the original tissue. Infection or haematoma delays wound healing by depressing collagen synthesis and increases wound tension.

22. (a) F.
    (b) F.
    (c) T.
    (d) F.
    (e) F.

Primary hyperparathyroidism is caused by overproduction of parathyroid hormone (PTH). In 90% of cases this is due to a single adenoma, or less commonly parathyroid hyperplasia or carcinoma. It may be asymptomatic or present with symptoms related to psychiatric, gastrointestinal or skeletal complications, but most often with urinary calculi. The diagnosis is confirmed by a persistently raised serum calcium. Secondary hyperparathyroidism results from PTH overproduction secondary to prolonged hypocalcium such as chronic renal failure, and serum calcium is usually normal. Tertiary hyperparathyroidism is caused by persistent PTH overproduction following removal of the hypocalcaemic stimulus resulting in hypercalcaemia.

23. (a) T.
    (b) F.
    (c) T.
    (d) F.
    (e) T.

Pituitary tumours account for 15% of all intracranial tumours and 75% are adenomas. Most begin in the pituitary fossa and this causes enlargement of the fossa which can be seen on X-ray. These tumours can present with signs of pituitary insufficiency such as hypothyroidism or less commonly, if the adenoma is secretory, Cushing's syndrome. If the tumour extends superiorly compression of the optic chiasma occurs. This produces variable visual disturbance, but classically bitemporal hemianopia. Signs and symptoms of raised intracranial pressure may also occur. Removal of the tumour is increasingly performed transphenoidally, avoiding the potential morbidity of frontal craniotomy. Large tumours may have to be removed by the latter method.

24. (a) T.
    (b) F.
    (c) T.
    (d) T.
    (e) F.

The incidence of melanoma is increasing at an alarming rate, especially in fair-skinned women living close to the equator. The most common type – superficial spreading melanoma – arises from a pre-existing naevus in only a third of cases. The best indicator of prognosis is the vertical tumour thickness. Melanomas are not radiosensitive and require surgical excision with a clearance margin proportional to the thickness.

25. (a) F.
    (b) T.
    (c) T.
    (d) T.
    (e) T.

Glucocorticoids occur naturally, secreted by the adrenal cortex, but are frequently given for their anti-inflammatory and immunosuppressive properties. The reduction in the inflammatory response may mask physical signs that are normally produced by the inflammatory response to disease and also risk fulminent infection in infectious conditions. Side-effects of steroid therapy include sodium retention (leading to hypertension or pulmonary oedema) and diabetes.

26. (a) T.
    (b) F.
    (c) T.
    (d) T.
    (e) F.

Autopsy studies suggest that over 90% of pulmonary emboli originate from lower limb and pelvic veins, but these often cannot be identified by venography or ultrasound. Other reported sources include mural thrombus from the right heart, pericatheter thrombus, paradoxical emboli which pass through a patent foramen ovale, and other material such as placental tissue and tumour. Most PEs are silent and not detected, but if untreated then approximately 30% of patients have a further fatal PE.

Diagnosis can be difficult and chest X-ray and electrocardiogram (ECG) changes are often non-specific. Technetium-99m perfusion scans may be abnormal for a number of reasons, but if normal a PE can be excluded. If the scan is abnormal a xenon ventilation scan is also performed and a ventilation–perfusion mismatch increases the probability of the diagnosis. Pulmonary angiography is invasive and associated with morbidity, but is probably the most accurate diagnostic test.

Full anticoagulation with heparin is commenced on diagnosis. Thrombolysis has shown promise in selected patients either directly by pulmonary artery catheter or systemically, but is still under evaluation. Following a massive PE, if the patient has survived the initial event, emergency pulmonary artery embolectomy should be undertaken if the facilities and expertise are available for immediate intervention.

27. (a) F.
    (b) F.
    (c) F.
    (d) F.
    (e) T.

Small bowel obstruction classically presents with vomiting followed by abdominal distension and pain, then finally constipation (which may not be a symptom at all, in contrast to left-sided large bowel obstruction). On examination the abdomen is distended, resonant to percussion and increased bowel sounds are present, unless very advanced, when bowel sounds may decrease due to secondary paralytic ileus. The commonest cause in adults is intra-abdominal adhesions from previous surgery, but care is needed not to miss a small femoral hernia in an overweight patient. X-rays reveal dilated bowel seen as a 'ladder pattern' centrally. Treatment is by resuscitation with intravenous fluids, nasogastric suction and analgesia, but early laparotomy is indicated to avoid bowel strangulation or perforation if symptoms do not settle rapidly.

28. (a) F.
    (b) F.
    (c) T.
    (d) F.
    (e) T.

Fractures involving the epiphyseal plates are serious as they may significantly alter the subsequent growth of the bone and interfere with function. Recognition of the injury, classification of its severity according to a system devised by Salter and Harris and account of the age of the child and how much further bone growth is expected must be taken into account. Many fractures involving the epiphysis can be managed by closed reduction. If the displacement is marked or closed reduction not possible, open reduction and fixation must be undertaken. Pathological fractures are less common in children, but can occur in areas of bony abnormality such as osteogenesis imperfecta and bone cysts.

Long bone fractures generally heal well and remodelling occurs so that residual deformity is unusual. However, rotational deformity does not correct well. Femoral shaft fractures are generally managed with traction on a Thomas splint. The traction can be adjusted to achieve reduction over the first few days.

29. (a) F.
    (b) F.
    (c) T.
    (d) T.
    (e) F.

Twisting of the sigmoid colon on its mesentery occurs when a long, redundant loop is associated with a narrow mesenteric base. It is commoner in races who take a high-fibre diet and in patients with chronic constipation. Twisting of the colon results in closed loop obstruction and, if severe, strangulation. The diagnosis is usually suspected clinically and confirmed by the classic X-ray appearance of two distended loops of bowel, separated by a thick wall, arising from the left iliac fossa and bulging up to the right upper quadrant. Suspected bowel strangulation or perforation requires urgent laparotomy, but many cases can be treated initially by sigmoidoscopy and flatus tube decompression. This allows elective treatment – sigmoid colectomy with primary anastomosis – to be performed later.

30. (a) T.
    (b) F.
    (c) T.
    (d) T.
    (e) F.

The possibility of occult intra-abdominal malignancy should be considered in patients with hepatomegaly or ascites. Advanced tumours may spread via the thoracic duct to the *left* supraclavicular fossa (Virchov's node). Carcinoma may also (uncommonly) spread transcoelomically to the umbilicus (Sister Mary Joseph's node). Campbell-de-Morgan spots are harmless manifestations of age.

31. (a) T.
    (b) F.
    (c) T.
    (d) F.
    (e) F.

Indications for tracheostomy include:
- Airway obstruction (foreign body, tumour, cord paralysis, severe facial injury when endotracheal intubation is not possible).
- Airway protection and toilet (e.g. in patient with depressed gag reflex).
- Prolonged mechanical ventilation.
- Major head and neck surgery, either to protect airway or if larynx has been removed.

Complications of tracheostomy include bleeding, obstruction of the tube, and damage to other structures. Airway stenosis can occur, especially if the cricoid is damaged (this is avoided if the trachea is opened below the second tracheal ring) or by prolonged overinflation of a cuffed tube resulting in pressure necrosis.

Although better performed under general anaesthesia, in some patients, especially those with respiratory obstruction, tracheostomy must be performed under local infiltration anaesthesia. On removal of the tracheostomy tube a dressing is placed over the hole which will close spontaneously, providing the airway is otherwise satisfactory.

32. (a) F.
    (b) T.
    (c) F.
    (d) F.
    (e) T.

Jaundiced patients require careful preparation prior to surgical or endoscopic biliary decompression. Rehydration (and possibly diuresis) is essential to prevent renal failure, and clotting deficiencies are corrected with parenteral vitamin K. A high protein diet might precipitate encephalopathy if hepatocellular failure is complicating the jaundice. Biliary stasis pre-disposes to infection, usually with Gram-negative organisms, and an appropriate antibiotic is administered intravenously. Whilst awaiting surgery, severe itching resulting from the jaundice may be relieved by antihistamines.

33. (a) T.
    (b) T.
    (c) T.
    (d) F.
    (e) T.
    Fallot's tetralogy comprises pulmonary valve stenosis and a large VSD. Valve stenosis results in right ventricular hypertrophy and the position of the VSD makes the aorta appear to override the right ventricle to complete the tetralogy originally described. A right-to-left shunt results, causing cyanosis and thus finger clubbing. Secondary polycythaemia is a consequence of cyanosis, increasing the risk of thromboembolic complications, especially cerebral. Treatment is invariably surgical correction. Severely affected infants may just have a shunt created between the aorta and the pulmonary artery (e.g. Blalock operation – subclavian artery to pulmonary artery) until fit enough for definitive correction. There is an increased risk of most congenital heart disorders with Down's syndrome.

34. (a) T.
    (b) F.
    (c) T.
    (d) F.
    (e) F.
    Carcinoma of the penis is relatively uncommon and, in the West, usually occurs in the glans of elderly uncircumcized men. The diagnosis is confirmed by biopsy and the lesion is a squamous cell carcinoma. It commonly spreads to the inguinal lymph nodes. Treatment involves circumcision to allow exposure of the tumour and local irradiation with iridium. If the tumour is advanced then partial or total amputation is required.

35. (a) F.
    (b) F.
    (c) T.
    (d) F.
    (e) T.

Fractures of the humeral shaft are generally treated non-operatively. The weight of the arm and forearm when supported in a collar and cuff usually provides enough traction to reduce the fracture. The fracture site may be supported by a plaster back slab or 'U' support to prevent movement and reduce pain as well as providing more weight for traction. A broad arm sling will not allow this method of traction to work as it supports the weight of the arm. If the elbow is injured it may be judged that internal fixation of the humerus would allow earlier mobilization of the arm and result in a better outcome for the elbow injury. Sometimes one of the bone ends 'button-holes' the triceps muscle and closed reduction is not possible. Under this circumstance, open reduction will be required.

The radial nerve, as it spirals around the posterior aspect of the humerus, is at greatest risk of injury resulting in wrist drop. It is rarely torn but usually contused and so surgical exploration is not usually undertaken.

Union usually occurs around 6 weeks for a spiral fracture and longer for a transverse fracture. Delayed or non-union of a transverse fracture may occur, especially if too much traction is applied.

36. (a) F.
    (b) T.
    (c) F.
    (d) T.
    (e) F.

Fractures of the radius and ulna often result in impairment of forearm function if reduction is not perfect. Closed manipulation and a plaster cast to prevent movement of the joint above and below the fracture site may be perfectly adequate, especially in children. However, if closed reduction is poor or if the reduction is lost in plaster open reduction and internal fixation should be undertaken. Some surgeons claim that the latter approach gives better functional results, but this view is not universally held.

Fracture of one cortex, a greenstick fracture, appears on the X-ray as a buckling of the cortex with angulation.

Reduction can usually be achieved by pressure under anaesthesia and is worth doing when obvious angulation has occurred. The condition is painful, and even in minor cases with minimal angulation a plaster back slab will make the child more comfortable.

Swelling after manipulation can be marked and pressure in the muscle compartments can rise above the arterial perfusion pressure. Usually, however, swelling occurs within the plaster and ischaemia of the arm occurs. Unless the plaster is released irreversible damage to the muscles and nerves of the arm result.

Fractures that are associated with overlying wounds need to be cleaned surgically and dead tissue removed. Internal fixation obviously carries the risk of infection and, although this may be required in some cases, is often best avoided if satisfactory reduction can be obtained and held without it.

37. (a) F.
    (b) F.
    (c) T.
    (d) T.
    (e) F.

Hodgkin's disease (adenolymphoma) usually presents with rubbery cervical lymphadenopathy. Splenomegally occurs in nearly half of cases and is frequently associated with systemic symptoms. Histologically, large binucleated cells (Reed–Sternberg cells) are seen with varying degrees of lymphocyte infiltration. Lymphocyte-predominant disease carries the best prognosis, then nodular sclerosing and mixed cellular, the lymphocyte depleted type being the most aggressive. Prognosis is also influenced by clinical stage but has generally improved with the advent of effective chemotherapy regimens and radiotherapy. Surgery is used mainly for diagnosis and staging, but even this role is diminishing due to modern imaging techniques.

38. (a) F.
    (b) T.
    (c) F.

(d) F.
(e) F.
Following tonsillectomy, any significant bleeding within the first few hours (primary or reactionary haemorrhage) requires return to the operating theatre and ligation of the bleeding point. Bleeding at 7–10 days (secondary haemorrhage) indicates infection and should be treated with antibiotics. Pain referred to the ear is quite common due to irritation of the glossopharyngeal nerve.

The value of one- or two-dose antibiotic prophylaxis for the procedure is debated, but certainly should not be continued for 7 days. There is no evidence that patients are more prone to bacterial chest infections after tonsillectomy (compare with splenectomy).

39. (a) F.
    (b) F.
    (c) F.
    (d) F.
    (e) T.
There are 25 000 new cases diagnosed and 19 000 deaths each year from colorectal cancer in the UK. There is no difference in incidence between the sexes. 25% of lesions occur in the right colon, 25% in the left colon and 50% in the rectum. The peak incidence is in 70–80 year olds. The commonest cause of large bowel obstruction is large bowel tumours. However, only 25–30% of patients with large bowel tumours present with obstruction, the rest have symptoms of change in bowel habit, bleeding and weight loss. Caecal tumours are unlikely to present with frank bleeding, but commonly cause anaemia, weight loss and general malaise. Local spread is mainly transversely, through the bowel wall. Hence, successful resection may be performed with only a few centimetres clearance of visible tumour, but should include a wide margin of neighbouring structures (e.g. mesorectum). Prognosis of lesions confined to the mucosa (Duke's stage A) is excellent, with a 5-year survival of over 95%. If the tumour has spread through the bowel wall (Duke's stage B), this is

reduced to about 70% and spread to lymph nodes (Duke's stage C) carries a 5-year survival of less than 30%.

40. (a) T.
    (b) F.
    (c) T.
    (d) F.
    (e) T.

Preservation of the knee joint gives a better chance of mobility as the prosthesis is lighter and problems of mechanical knee joints are avoided. Failure of the amputation to heal may result in further amputation at a higher level and so it is important to determine whether the blood supply to the below-knee skin is adequate to heal. This is usually based on clinical impression, although transcutaneous oxygen tension can be used. Between 10% and 20% of below-knee amputations fail to heal and have to be revised.

Early mobility is important to preserve joint mobility and muscle tone. The stump takes time to heal and then mature before a definitive prosthesis can be fitted. In the early stages a patient can often walk using a pneumatic post-amputation mobility (PAM) aid from around day 5–7 after surgery.

As the operation involves resection of bone antibiotics should be given prior to surgery to ensure adequate levels at the time of the procedure. The cause of phantom limb pain is unknown. Transcutaneous nerve stimulation, drugs such as carbamazepine and prolonged epidural infusion of local anaesthetic are claimed to help. Repeated amputation is rarely helpful.

41. (a) F.
    (b) T.
    (c) T.
    (d) T.
    (e) T.

Such an injury can avulse the brachial plexus as well as cause severe head, neck and shoulder injuries. The more proximal the injury the worse the prognosis for recovery and if the pre-ganglionic nerve roots have been avulsed then no recovery occurs. Damage to the sympathetic chain occurs with proximal root lesions and so is an indicator of poor prognosis. Fractures of the transverse processes, too, can occur and imply severe injury.

Damage to the C5 and C6 roots will cause paralysis of the abductors and external rotators of the shoulder and the forearm supinators are paralysed. The arm is held in the characteristic position, adducted at the shoulder, extended at the elbow, pronated and flexed at the wrist ('the waiter's tip position').

If complete avulsion has occurred the only chance of recovery is microsurgical repair by a specialist as soon as the general condition of the patient allows. Some surgeons feel that the results of this are not worthwhile. If the patient is left with a flaccid senseless arm many will opt for amputation through the humerus.

42. (a) T.
    (b) F.
    (c) T.
    (d) T.
    (e) F.

Hypertension is the usual finding but hypotensive episodes occur. Urinary catecholamine metabolites such as VMA are elevated. The diagnosis can be confirmed using an adrenergic blocker (phentolamine) which will produce hypotension in the absence of a phaechromocytoma. This can be dangerous and imaging with CT and magnetic resonance imaging (MRI) will usually locate the tumour, 10% of which are extra-adrenal, 10% malignant and 10% bilateral.

43. (a) T.
    (b) F.
    (c) F.
    (d) T.
    (e) F.

At least 1% of the adult population have a leg ulcer and approximately 80% of these patients have venous disease.

The male/female ratio is about 3:1, but venous ulcers are the commonest cause of leg ulceration in men. Venous obstruction or damage to valves resulting from a DVT can result in venous ulceration, which may not present for years after the initial event.

There is often an underlying, surgically correctable venous problem when the patient presents with an ulcer. It depends on the condition of the patient and the facilities available, but there is no reason to postpone surgical interventions as correction of the underlying problem may speed up ulcer healing when combined with non-surgical treatments.

Local dressing should provide an ideal environment for healing and be practical. There is little objective evidence to support the choice of dressing, but hydrocolloids are widely used. They are absorbent and gas-permeable and provide a good environment for healing. Dry dressings tend to require more regular changing as they become saturated with exudate and this may damage new epithelium. Semipermeable membranes provide a good healing environment but are often impractical. Whatever local dressing is used, adequate compression or correction of the underlying venous disease is also necessary.

Skin grafting (split skin or pinch grafts) may speed up the healing of a large ulcer, but the recurrence rate is high unless the underlying problem is corrected. Removal of dead tissue from around an ulcer is necessary, but radical excision of the ulcer is rarely practised although it has been reported.

44. (a) F.
    (b) T.
    (c) T.
    (d) T.
    (e) T.

Anorectal anomalies are the most frequent congenital abnormality of the gut occurring in one in 3000–4000 live births. There is an increased risk of other congenital abnormalities, especially of the upper renal tract which will be found in 25% and ultrasound of the renal tract must be performed to identify these.

Careful inspection of the anus must be performed in a child that has not passed meconium. A bulging membrane may be discovered or an anal stenosis. The rectum may pass through the pelvic floor, but end blindly in a low imperforate anus. If the rectum fails to pass through the pelvic floor the lesion is high. Fistulas may be found, often in the midline with imperforate anus. Rarely, the rectum may fail to develop (rectal agenesis). The level of obstruction can be determined by a plain X-ray taken with the baby inverted and air can be seen in the terminal part of the gut. This test has limited value as time must be allowed for the passage of air through the gut after delivery, and as the baby often cries and struggles the level can be difficult to assess.

Low lesions may be treated by a cut-back operation, but high lesions require colostomy and a pull-through procedure when the child is older.

45. (a) T.
    (b) F.
    (c) F.
    (d) T.
    (e) F.

Venous ulcers may be due to deep venous insufficiency following DVT or superficial venous hypertension associated with varicose veins. They commonly occur above the medial malleolus. Infected ulcers associated with cellulitis should be treated with oral antibiotics but, once clean, a simple non-adherent dressing is followed by compression bandaging and advice to elevate the limb. Most ulcers will heal with proper compression and elevation. Once healed, the underlying cause should be sought with duplex ultrasound or venography and treated surgically if appropriate. Anticoagulants are prescribed for acute DVT, but not for chronic venous ulcers.

46. (a) F.
    (b) T.
    (c) T.
    (d) F.
    (e) F.

Inguinal hernias seen in children are indirect, due to a patent processus vaginalis, and should be repaired as strangulation is a real risk. Excision of the sac at the deep ring (herniotomy) is all that is required. Congenital indirect sacs may be present for many years and only present with a hernia in adulthood. Complete scrotal hernias have the testis in the lower part of the sac. Indirect hernias tend to take an oblique passage from deep to external ring and are controllable by finger pressure over the deep ring. Direct hernias tend to occur in elderly men due to a weakness of the posterior inguinal wall. They protrude at right angles to the groin skin. However, clinical differences may be blurred and the only certain method of diagnosis is at operation. Inguinal hernias occur in women, but are less common due to the vestigial nature of the inguinal canal. Up to 30% of inguinal hernias may be bilateral.

47. (a) F.
    (b) T.
    (c) F.
    (d) T.
    (e) T.

The differential diagnosis is between a parotid swelling (pleomorphic adenoma most commonly, or an adenolymphoma or carcinoma), lymphadenopathy or a lesion of the skin or subcutaneous tissue. If it is not possible to determine the diagnosis, FNAC may help. Facial nerve palsy suggests infiltration by malignancy. Excision biopsy is unacceptable because if the lump is a pleomorphic adenoma recurrence will be very likely and the risk of developing a salivary fistula is high by this approach.

If a pleomorphic adenoma is suspected a superficial parotidectomy is the best treatment. If the lesion is an enlarged lymph node which persists then malignancy or lymphoma need to be excluded either by FNAC or by removal and histological examination.

48. (a) F.
    (b) F.
    (c) F.
    (d) T.
    (e) F.

Arterial and venous injury is a relatively uncommon, but if missed disastrous, complication of long bone fracture. Recording of pedal pulses at the time of admission of a patient who may be very unwell, hypotensive and have other injuries is often inaccurate. If there is doubt recording of the ankle systolic blood pressure using Doppler ultrasound is helpful. Conversely, significant intimal injuries to an artery may have occurred but the artery remains patent at first, occluding several hours later.

Lack of pulsatile blood flow in an artery implies significant injury, not spasm, and must be treated as such. If the patient is stable angiography should be obtained, but often the patient is actively bleeding and urgent surgical exploration and per-operative angiography should be undertaken. Temporary shunts provide time for fractured bones to be fixed and suitable vein for bypass to be harvested. Whenever possible significant venous injuries should be repaired rather than ligated as chronic venous insufficiency may result. The general condition of the patient must be taken into account when planning time-consuming repairs.

49. (a) T.
    (b) T.
    (c) F.
    (d) T.
    (e) F.

Squamous cell carcinoma (SCC) is more aggressive than basal cell carcinoma and metastasizes to regional lymph nodes. The classical appearance is as above but may be a fleshy, fungating tumour. The centre of such tumours undergoes necrosis to produce the characteristic ulcer. SCC is pre-disposed to by ultraviolet radiation but may also result from chronic skin inflammation in chronic sinuses and scars in irradiated skin and ulcers (Marjolin's ulcers). Chemical irritation with dyes, tar and soot also causes SCC. The first industrial cancer described was SCC of the scrotum in chimney sweeps of the 18th century. Treatment is by excision and grafting with block dissection of involved nodes.

50. (a) T.
    (b) F.
    (c) T.
    (d) F.
    (e) T.

Most anal fissures are of unknown aetiology, but are probably due to tearing of the anal skin by hard faeces. A minority are associated with proctitis or Crohn's disease. Symptoms are severe pain on defaecation and sometimes bleeding or perianal irritation. On examination, the fissure is usually seen in the midline posteriorly, but it is often impossible to examine the anus properly due to intense pain and spasm. Oedematous anal skin at the external aspect of the fissure ('sentinal pile') may, however, be present. Fissures may heal spontaneously and symptomatic relief with local anaesthetic gel is all that is required. If conservative management fails, examination under anaesthetic is indicated to confirm the diagnosis. Most surgeons perform an anal stretch to relieve spasm but this risks recurrence of symptoms or incontinence. A lateral cutaneous sphincterotomy, dividing the most superficial fibres of the internal sphincter, is probably more effective and safer.

ANSWERS TO PAPER 5

1. (a) T.
   (b) T.
   (c) F.
   (d) F.
   (e) T.
   This patient is most likely to be suffering from advanced malignancy. After confirmation of multiple liver metastases by ultrasound screening, a liver biopsy is useful to achieve a histological diagnosis. This excludes benign conditions such as multiple abscesses or tumours that may respond to chemotherapy, especially lymphoma. The most likely cause, however, is an adenocarcinoma from the gut or pancreas and management is palliative. A prolonged 'hunt the primary' is of no benefit and the best place to be is usually at home with adequate support, or in a hospice when death is imminent and symptoms cannot be controlled. Palliative measures include analgesics, antiemetics, antipruritics, and steroids. Radiotherapy is useful for relieving pain caused by liver secondaries.

2. (a) F.
   (b) F.
   (c) T.
   (d) F.
   (e) T.
   Testicular torsion is the commonest cause of a child or young man presenting with an acutely painful, swollen testicle. Epididymo-orchitis is rare. The underlying cause of torsion is a high insertion of the tunica vaginalis, allowing the testicle to twist. The abnormality is usually bilateral and the testicles tend to lie horizontally. The diagnosis cannot safely be excluded by clinical examination

and in most cases urgent surgical exploration is indicated. Doppler ultrasound can be used to pick up a signal from the testicular artery which, if present, is claimed to make the diagnosis of torsion unlikely. However, some testicles undergo repeated episodes of torsion and spontaneous derotation and so surgical exploration is still usually necessary to exclude this possibility. Should torsion be confirmed, bilateral fixation should be performed. If presentation or exploration is delayed, a necrotic testicle may need to be excised. To reduce this risk, attempts at immediate manual detorsion have been advocated, but in practice this is of little value and urgent surgical exploration is the priority.

3. (a) F.
   (b) T.
   (c) F.
   (d) T.
   (e) F.

Two-thirds of bone secondaries arise from the breast or prostate. Other sources include thyroid, kidney, bronchus, testicle, and occasionally gut and bladder. Osteolytic secondaries such as occur from the breast are more common than osteosclerotic lesions which often originate from the prostate. Despite extensive investigation, in around 10% of cases the primary tumour will not be found. In most cases the management will not be altered, although lymphoma deposits should be identified as chemotherapy may be indicated.

Patients may present with pain, pathological fractures or signs of compression as in the vertebral column. Some lesions are found incidentally on X-ray. Treatment is analgesia and anti-inflammatories. Internal fixation is often very effective, providing the general health of the patient allows surgery. It prevents movement at the fracture site and so reduces pain as well as restoring some function. Radiotherapy locally to the secondary is effective at reducing pain and may be combined with internal fixation.

ANSWERS TO PAPER FIVE 181

4. (a) F.
   (b) F.
   (c) T.
   (d) T.
   (e) F.

   In this age group a breast lump is most likely to be a fibroadenoma. Carcinoma is rare but no lump should be ignored. FNAC may confirm the diagnosis and exclude a simple cyst. Most surgeons prefer to remove all breast lumps and many women request excision, but some contend that fibroadenoma confidently diagnosed on FNAC may be left. Mammography is likely to be unhelpful in young women. The low-dose contraceptive pill is not known to increase the risk of breast lump.

5. (a) F.
   (b) F.
   (c) F.
   (d) T.
   (e) T.

   Laparoscopic techniques have reduced the hospital stay and discomfort of most patients having cholecystectomy, but the procedure has not changed the indications for surgery. The risk of carcinoma of the gallbladder is too small to justify removal of asymptomatic gallstones. Patients with a good history of gallstone symptoms (biliary colic, acute cholecystisis) require cholecystectomy and this can now usually be achieved laparoscopically, although the conversion rate to an open procedure is high in patients with acute inflammation. Fatty food intolerance is a common symptom in middle-aged women and gallstones are often present, but a causal relationship has not been established and many continue to complain of identical symptoms after an ill-advised cholecystectomy. The patient in (b) requires an urgent ERCP and sphincterotomy.

6. (a) T.
   (b) F.
   (c) T.

(d) T.
(e) T.

Approximately 50% of intracranial tumours are metastases from sites such as the bronchus and breast. Patients with intracranial tumours may present with signs and symptoms of raised intracranial pressure such as headache, vomiting, papilloedema, focal neurological signs, hydrocephalus or focal epilepsy. The presentation of epilepsy in an adult should raise the suspicion of an intracranial tumour.

Meningiomas make up about 20% of intracranial tumours, but tend to be well defined, 90% are supratentorial and so surgical removal is often possible and is the best treatment option. The tumour may cause erosion of the overlying skull and be apparent on X-ray. Up to 20% of meningiomas may recur however, often due to incomplete removal.

7. (a) T.
   (b) F.
   (c) T.
   (d) F.
   (e) F.

Heart failure is a common cause of limb swelling but does not result in unilateral oedema which is more likely caused by venous obstruction (following thrombosis or external compression, e.g. a pelvic mass), lymphatic failure due to damage from repeated infection, obstruction due to malignancy, or congenital abnormalities. Congenital lymphatic hypoplasia (Milroy's disease) often does not present until adulthood and is often precipitated by a minor injury or infection.

Depending on the cause of the oedema and the degree of distress caused, most treatment is conservative and involves limb elevation, compression stockings, intermittent compression devices and aggressive treatment of infection. Venous bypass surgery for obliterated major veins is only for advanced cases and, although lymphovenous bypass is very occasionally performed, debulking procedures are only undertaken for the most extreme conditions.

8. (a) T.
   (b) T.
   (c) F.
   (d) T.
   (e) F.

A transplanted organ risks rejection by the recipient's immune system and ABO incompatability results in hyperacute (immediate) rejection. The HLA histocompatibility antigens are less important but the closer the match the better the chances of success. With modern immunosuppressive drugs, however, a total match is not necessary. Long-term immunosuppressive therapy risks opportunistic infections and malignancy. Graft survival at 5 years depends on haplotype matching, with genetically identical siblings providing the best results. Overall graft survival on good units is now over 70%.

9. (a) F.
   (b) F.
   (c) T.
   (d) T.
   (e) F.

In patients who present with minor neurological events, carotid artery disease will be the cause in less then 20% and they should be reviewed by a neurologist. Carotid angiography is invasive and is associated with morbidity; thus it is not indicated in the first instance. Carotid duplex scanning is safe and accurate and is the ideal initial investigation for these patients.

Even in patients with proven carotid disease anticoagulation has no role. In patients with minor (<30%), symptomatic stenoses the risk of a subsequent major stroke is small (2% or less over 2 years) and there is good evidence that aspirin is the best treatment.

10. (a) F.
    (b) T.
    (c) F.
    (d) F.
    (e) T.

Haemorrhoidectomy is indicated for very large, third-degree (prolapsed) or strangulated piles. The operation is painful and may be complicated by urinary retention, reactionary haemorrhage or anal stenosis if too much anal skin is excised. Outpatient treatments have therefore taken over for most patients. Patients should be encouraged to take a high-fibre diet so that they do not have to strain at stool. Injection sclerotherapy is effective for first-degree (non-prolapsing) haemorrhoids and rubber-band ligation for larger (second-degree) piles, but banding should not be used below the dentate line as this is very painful. Other effective treatments include cryotherapy (freezing) or laser coagulation. Haemorrhoids may be associated with anal spasm, especially in young men, but it remains controversial whether relief with an anal stretch is effective. Certainly, recurrence rates are high and it should never be performed in the elderly as incontinence is common.

11. (a) T.
    (b) T.
    (c) F.
    (d) T.
    (e) T.

Chronic osteomyelitis may follow compound fractures, surgical intervention, acute osteomyelitis or, rarely, presents as a primary event, especially if the infecting organism is unusual (e.g. tubercle). The pressure of the pus in the acute stages may result in bone necrosis. The dead bone may subsequently be discharged or form a sequestrum. Surrounding bone may become osteosclerotic so that the X-ray appearance is of rarefaction surrounded by sclerosis and dead bone. The infection may apparently settle only to flare up again, sometimes years later. Treatment is by antibiotics and, if possible, removal of the dead and infected tissue. Sometimes abscess cavities may be seen in the metaphysis (Brodie's abscess). These may present with episodic pain and require surgical drainage.

12. (a) T.
    (b) F.

(c) T.
(d) T.
(e) F.

Posterior urethral valves are the commonest cause of lower-urinary-tract obstruction in boys. Diagnosis may be suspected on antenatal ultrasound scans which reveal dilated kidneys and a distended bladder. In the early post-natal period the child may not pass urine or has a feeble stream and ultrasound demonstrates an enlarged bladder and dilated upper renal tract. If the diagnosis is missed the child may present late with recurrent urinary-tract infections or renal failure.

Diagnosis can be confirmed on a micturating cystourethrogram. The valves prevent the passage of urine, but a fine-bore tube can be passed retrogradely. This should only be done by an experienced paediatrician. Treatment is endoscopic ablation of the valves.

13. (a) F.
    (b) T.
    (c) T.
    (d) F.
    (e) F.

Haemorrhoids (piles) are prolapses of the anal cushions that are responsible for fine continence and classically occur at '3, 7 and 11 o'clock' (with '12 o'clock' anterior). They contain branches of the superior rectal arteries and veins but are *not* varicose veins. Prolapse probably occurs due to increased rectal pressure upon straining at stool, and thus a high-fibre diet is protective. Pregnancy increases pelvic vasculature, makes tissues more lax and causes venous congestion, so piles are common. Haemorrhoids commonly present with bleeding or the sensation of prolapse on defaecation, which may be associated with mucous discharge and pruritis ani. Internal haemorrhoids are not usually palpable but can be viewed with a proctoscope. Prolapsed piles may strangulate and produce acute, severe pain.

14. (a) T.
    (b) F.
    (c) T.
    (d) F.
    (e) T.

Distinction of vasculogenic claudication from arthritis and neurological claudication (due to spinal canal stenosis) can be difficult. A claudicant with peripheral vascular disease usually has a moderate reduction in ankle systolic blood pressure at rest compared to brachial artery pressure. On exercise the pressure will fall and take several minutes to return to the resting level. In a subject without vascular disease ankle blood pressure does not fall.

Only 10–15% of patients will progress to limb-threatening ischaemia, which must be remembered when planning treatment. Cessation of smoking will reduce overall cardiovascular mortality rate, and there is evidence to suggest it will also improve walking. Weight reduction likewise increases the distance that patients can walk. Although there are a number of drugs which have a variety of effects on the circulation (vasoactive), none has been consistently shown to be of objective benefit.

15. (a) F.
    (b) T.
    (c) F.
    (d) F.
    (e) F.

In the patient described, mesenteric embolus should always be considered. Classically, in the early stages (before bowel necrosis) pain is severe but abdominal signs are minimal. If other causes can be eliminated, laparotomy may be indicated to attempt revascularization before necrosis occurs. High white-cell count, acidosis and impaired renal function suggest severe ischaemia or necrosis. Necrotic bowel may cause the serum amylase to rise. Early resuscitation to correct hypovolaemia is essential, but the patient's general condition continues to deteriorate until the necrotic bowel has been excised. Full resuscitation is impossible unless the necrotic bowel is excised, which is a priority. In most cases, extensive bowel necrosis is seen at laparotomy with a very high associated mortality. Even if embolectomy is successful, reperfusion of a large segment of ischaemic gut incites a severe systemic reaction, risking cardiac arrest, renal failure and Adult Respiratory Distress Syndrome (ARDS). Thus, mortality remains high.

16. (a) F.
    (b) T.
    (c) T.
    (d) T.
    (e) F.

RA is a generalized inflammatory condition primarily affecting the synovium of joints and tendons. It is associated with antibodies to IgG and rheumatoid factors, but they are non-specific and are not elevated in 20% of cases. The disease can progress insidiously or be episodic and associated with severe systemic illness. Vasculitis can affect the heart, kidney, lung, brain and extremities. Lymphadenopathy is very common; subcutaneous nodules consisting of a necrotic centre surrounded by inflammatory cells can be found especially over the dorsal aspect of the forearm.

Initial treatment includes analgesia and anti-inflammatory agents. Intra-articular steroids are often used but, if repeated frequently, may result in a symptomless deterioration of the joint. Systemic steroids are occasionally used, particularly while waiting for other agents such as penicillamine or gold to achieve their benefit, but care is needed to monitor the side-effects. Immunosuppressive drugs such as cyclophosphamide or azothiaprine can be as effective. Synovectomy may help, and joint replacement or arthrodesis is required if destruction is advanced.

17. (a) F.
    (b) T.
    (c) F.
    (d) F.
    (e) T.

Colonic carcinomas more commonly present with the passage of altered blood over a longer time-scale. Procto-sigmoidoscopy is indicated (mainly to exclude haemorrhoids), but the most likely diagnoses are diverticulosis or angiodysplasia of the colon. Diverticular bleeding is usually self-limiting, but angiodyspastic bleeding may be persistent or recurrent. Barium enema is unlikely to locate the bleeding point and is rarely helpful in the emergency situation. Mesenteric angiography is helpful if bleeding continues, but is useless when bleeding has stopped. Angiography or colonoscopy may isolate an angiodysplastic bleed, but sometimes laparotomy is needed and on-table panendoscopy of the gut is performed. The right colon is the commonest site for angiodyspasias.

18. (a) T.
    (b) F.
    (c) F.
    (d) F.
    (e) T.

ERCP is performed via a flexible, side-viewing endoscope and can be combined with sphincterotomy and stone extraction to clear the common bile duct of gallstones or with stenting of biliary tumours. Potential complications include bleeding, perforation, pancreatitis and biliary sepsis, but it is now a safe procedure with a mortality of less than 1%. Jaundiced patients should undergo an ultrasound scan first however, and ERCP should only be performed if dilated bile ducts are seen and obstructive jaundice suggested. Patients with pancreatitis and evidence of a gallstone impacted in the common bile duct may benefit from early ERCP and sphincterotomy.

19. (a) F.
    (b) T.
    (c) F.
    (d) F.
    (e) T.

For intra-arterial angiography a catheter is placed, if possible, via the femoral artery on the symptomatic side so that if damage or atheromatous embolization occur it will be in the leg which is being considered for treatment. If the femoral artery is completely occluded the opposite side can be used. Failing that, the choice is translumbar puncture of the aorta, or the brachial artery (which is small and prone to injury) or an IV-DSA. Puncture of the artery with a hollow needle, placement of a flexible guidewire through it so that it can be removed and catheter advancement over the guidewire was developed by Seldinger.

Digital subtraction techniques store a control picture which is then subtracted from subsequent films. This will allow less contrast to be used if an intra-arterial injection of contrast is made. In theory, intravenous injection of contrast should be sufficient to obtain an arteriogram. In practice, large volumes of contrast via a central venous line have to delivered rapidly to obtain acceptable images and this can cause problems in patients with ischaemic heart disease who cannot cope with a sudden volume load. As no foreign material is being implanted, antibiotics are not routinely given.

20. (a) F.
    (b) F.
    (c) T.
    (d) T.
    (e) F.

TPN is given intravenously, usually via a central line into a large vein. It is indicated for the nutritional support of severely ill patients, especially those who cannot absorb enteral feeds and are very catabolic due to major surgery, trauma, sepsis or organ failure. It is especially valuable in patients with high-output small bowel fistulas. It should be attempted to match the feed to the net requirements of the patient, but should include calories, with a large proportion given as fat, protein, essential fatty acids, vitamins and trace elements. There is little evidence that routine pre-operative use of TPN reduces morbidity of major surgery.

21. (a) F.
    (b) F.

(c) F.
(d) F.
(e) T.

A cystic hygroma is a multi-loculated cystic mass which represents a developmental abnormality of the lymphatic system and is apparent at birth or within the first few years of life. It is benign and most often occurs in the base of the posterior triangle of the neck, although it can extend into the chest or up to the mouth. It should not be confused with a thyroglossal cyst which is found in the midline of the neck anteriorly and moves up when the tongue is stuck out. Treatment is surgical excision.

22. (a) T.
    (b) T.
    (c) F.
    (d) T.
    (e) F.

NEC is a diffuse or focal ulceration of the small and large bowel and is a frequent cause of intestinal perforation in the neonate. It occurs in 1–2% of premature babies, but other than prematurity the aetiology is unknown. Infection does not seem to be the primary event, but usually becomes a major feature of the disease.

The baby develops abdominal distension, vomiting and blood in the stool during the first few days of life. Diagnosis is supported by plain abdominal X-ray which shows intramural gas in the bowel. Treatment is to withhold enteral feeds, intravenous fluids and antibiotics. If progression continues it may be necessary to resect the involved segments of bowel with the formation of temporary stomas. The overall survival is 70–80%.

23. (a) T.
    (b) F.
    (c) T.
    (d) F.
    (e) T.

Pruritis ani may result from mucous discharge from the anus due to fissure, fistula, haemorrhoids or proctitis, or be secondary to a vaginal discharge (candidiasis or trichomonas) or, uncommonly, due to threadworm infection. It is often idiopathic. On examination, the perianal skin appears red, excoriated and oedematous. Treatment is to eradicate any underlying cause, then break the 'vicious circle' of itching–scratching–excoriation. Moistened cotton wool or moist toilet tissue should replace conventional tissue to reduce perianal trauma. The anus should be dried thoroughly after washing and overheating and sweating (e.g. caused by tight nylon underwear) should be avoided. Strong topical steroids may damage the skin. A short course of 1% hydrocortisone may bring symptomatic relief, but treatment should be directed at the underlying cause of irritation. Zinc and castor oil cream is soothing and non-irritant when excoriation is severe.

24. (a) F.
    (b) T.
    (c) F.
    (d) F.
    (e) T.
    Smoking doubles the risk of developing pancreatic carcinoma. High alcohol intake is associated with pancreatic carcinoma, although whether this is a direct effect of the alcohol is not established. There is also a positive relationship with diabetes mellitus. There is no evidence that inflammatory conditions of the pancreas predispose to malignancy. Pain is the presenting complaint in 50–80%, jaundice in 10–30% and weight loss is apparent in 90% of cases. The majority of patients are dead within 6 months of presenting. Tumours of the ampulla present earlier with jaundice and, therefore, have a 5-year survival rate of 30–50% after resection.

25. (a) F.
    (b) T.
    (c) F.
    (d) F.
    (e) T.
    Ureteric calculi may cause very severe pain (colic), but

pyrexia suggests associated infection. Opiates, particularly pethidine, are traditionally given, but non-steroid anti-inflammatory drugs (NSAIDs) such as diclofenac are also effective. A high fluid intake is effective in preventing the formation of recurrent stones after the acute attack, but is ineffective in the acute stages, may increase pain and could theoretically exacerbate renal damage. 90% of ureteric calculi are seen on a plain X-ray and an IVU (if performed before the stone has passed) is diagnostic.

26. (a) F.
    (b) T.
    (c) T.
    (d) T.
    (e) F.

AS is a chronic inflammatory condition affecting the spine and sacroiliac joints. Males are most frequently affected and there is a strong association with HLA-B27. It usually presents in young men between 15 and 30 years of age as stiffness and pain in the sacroiliac region and lumbar spine. The condition involves inflammation, fibrosis and ossification. It affects fibrosseous joints such as the intervertebral discs and small joints such as the vertebral facet and sacroiliac joints. The result is pain, stiffness, deformity and loss of function. The earliest X-ray changes are erosions of the sacroiliac joints, but as ossification progresses this becomes visible and the vertebral column takes on the classic appearance of a 'Bamboo spine'. At first there is a loss of spinal movement and lumbar lordosis. Progressive loss of extension of the spine causes marked deformity and respiratory function may be impaired due to the deformity of the thoracic spine and also due to stiffness of the costovertebral joints.

Treatment is reduction of pain with analgesics and anti-inflammatory drugs and attempts to reduce subsequent deformity with physiotherapy. In established severe deformity, osteotomy of the spine may have to be undertaken.

ANSWERS TO PAPER FIVE

27. (a) T.
    (b) F.
    (c) T.
    (d) T.
    (e) F.
    An anal fissure usually arises after spontaneous discharge of a perianal abscess, but may complicate Crohn's disease, proctitis or tuberculosis. Symptoms are of soreness, discharge, irritation and pruritis ani. Goodsall's rule dictates that anterior fistulas communicate directly with the anal canal, whereas posterior fistulas enter the anus in the midline posteriorly, taking a 'horseshoe' shaped path. Anal fistulas rarely heal spontaneously and surgical intervention is necessary. 'Low' fistulas merely require laying open, but complex, high fistulas need specialist evaluation and management.

28. (a) T.
    (b) T.
    (c) F.
    (d) F.
    (e) F.
    Stones most commonly cause symptoms of obstruction in the submandibular gland and this may be noticed when salivating. If the stone is palpable in the submandibular duct it may be possible to remove it through the floor of the mouth. If the gland has become enlarged due to the obstruction or secondary infection then the gland and duct should be removed. Salivary calculi do not impose an increased risk of malignancy and are not usually associated with abnormal calcium metabolism.

29. (a) T.
    (b) T.
    (c) F.
    (d) F.
    (e) T.
    Below the knee the long saphenous vein, used *in situ* with the valves destroyed and the branches ligated or reversed,

gives superior results to prosthetic material such as Dacron or polytetrafluoroethylene (PTFE). Even with vein, patency rates at 1 year vary between 80% and 90% in the best series. Immediate or early (6 weeks) graft failure is usually due to technical errors or the selection of the wrong level of bypass. During the first year up to 30% of vein grafts develop stenoses due to intimal hyperplasia and, if not treated, these may go on to graft occlusion. After 1–2 years failed grafts are increasingly due to progression of atheroma. The effects of aspirin on graft patency are debatable and probably only marginal, but aspirin produces a significant reduction in overall cardiovascular mortality in patients with peripheral vascular disease.

30. (a) F.
    (b) F.
    (c) F.
    (d) F.
    (e) T.

IBS is being increasingly diagnosed as a cause of chronic abdominal symptoms for which no anatomical cause can be found. Symptoms vary, but colicky abdominal pain, post-prandial bloating, borborygmi with intermittent constipation and diarrhoea are typical. It is important to exclude serious pathology such as inflammatory bowel disease or malignancy before diagnosing IBS. IBS is a functional bowel disorder, but no underlying cause has been identified. It tends to be exacerbated by stress, major life traumas and certain foods. Treatment is by reassurance, stress avoidance, regular meals and a high-fibre diet. Thus a change in life-style often helps. Severe colicky pain may be controlled by antispasmodics. The condition is usually self-limiting.

31. (a) T.
    (b) T.
    (c) T.
    (d) F.
    (e) T.

Associated risk factors for bladder tumours include

nitrophenols (used in a number of industries), smoking and schistosomiasis. Transitional cell carcinoma is the most common, but squamous metaplasia can occur and adenocarcinomas can occur in the urachal remnants.

The tumours are staged according to the TMN (Tumours, Metastases, Nodes) classification: Ta, non-invasive (not through basement membrane); T1, not through lamina propria; T2, invasion of the superficial muscle; T3, invasion of the deep muscle; and T4, extravesical spread. N refers to the involvement of lymph nodes which is very difficult to assess and M to the presence of metastases. T1 tumours are treated by resection with the resectoscope. T3 tumours are usually treated by radiotherapy and total cystectomy.

32. (a) T.
    (b) F.
    (c) T.
    (d) F.
    (e) T.

In a young child, bone infection may follow direct infection via a wound, but usually bacteria are blood borne from another focus such as the ear, throat or a remote abscess. *Staphylococci* are commonly implicated, but other organisms such as *Pneumococci* and *Haemophili* can be responsible. The blood-borne bacteria settle in the metaphysis and infection can spread under the periosteum, along the medullary cavities or into a joint if the metaphysis is intra-articular. The epiphysis tends to act as a barrier to the spread of infection.

There is often a preceding history of a minor injury to the area. This can make diagnosis difficult, and if the symptoms seem out of proportion to the injury infection should be considered. Areas of redness and localized tenderness, together with refusal to use the limb are very suspicious, but often in the early stages no X-ray changes are apparent. Isotope bone scans or magnetic resonance imaging may reveal changes earlier. If the diagnosis remains in doubt, or there is no response to antibiotics, it is necessary to drain the infection either by incising the periosteum or by drilling the cortex of the bone. This can reduce pain by relieving the pressure and also allows direct identification of the causative organism.

33. (a) F.
    (b) T.
    (c) T.
    (d) T.
    (e) F.

Peritonitis commonly follows a perforated viscus. Symptoms are pain (worse on movement) and vomiting. On examination, the patient is tachycardic, pyrexial, hypotensive, peripherally shut down and clammy. The patient lies still, with the abdomen held rigidly. The abdomen is tender (with rebound and guarding) and bowel sounds are absent.

34. (a) T.
    (b) T.
    (c) T.
    (d) F.
    (e) F.

All patients with haematemesis require hospital admission as the condition is potentially life-threatening. Resuscitation is the priority with oxygen, intravenous fluids and blood. Next, endoscopy should be performed to identify the source of bleeding – this is most likely peptic ulceration or erosion. Oesophageal varices should always be considered but are uncommon, especially in elderly patients. Bleeding stops spontaneously in most patients but this may be assisted by diathermy, laser or alcohol or adrenaline injection coagulation via the endoscope. Should bleeding continue, surgical intervention is required to under-run the ulcer. In young patients, the threshold for surgery is high (e.g. >6–8 units blood transfused or a second rebleed), but elderly patients can tolerate less cardiovascular instability and so early surgery is advised (e.g. >4 units of blood transfused, first rebleed).

35. (a) F.
    (b) F.
    (c) F.
    (d) T.
    (e) F.

Once a Dacron graft has been in place for 2–3 days it becomes covered with a layer of platelets and fibrin (pseudointima) and there is no need to give prophylactic antibiotics unless the graft is exposed during the procedure. Blood flow through aortic grafts is high and patency rates excellent, so anticoagulation is not routinely employed. Follow-up of Dacron grafts implanted over 25 years previously has failed to reveal any significant material degradation. Most patients with aneurysms are elderly and the implanted graft will easily last the rest of their life.

Late complications are uncommon. It is estimated that around 3% of patients will develop further aneurysms, either true aneurysms above or below the graft or false aneurysms at the anastomoses, over 20 years. One of the most serious complications is the development of a fistula between the graft/aortic anastomoses and the bowel, most commonly the duodenum, the fourth part of which lies directly over the anastomosis. This is associated with graft infection. The patient may have a massive haematemesis, but often presents with a series of small 'herald' bleeds, and the diagnosis should always be considered in a patient who has had an aneurysm repair. Treatment usually requires removal of the graft and oversewing of the aortic stump, repair of the duodenum and restoration of blood supply to the lower torso by an axillobifemoral bypass. This carries a high operative mortality. Some surgeons will replace the aortic graft with an antibiotic-impregnated graft if infection is not overt.

36. (a) F.
    (b) T.
    (c) T.
    (d) T.
    (e) T.

Strangulation of a hernia implies that the blood supply to the hernial contents has become impaired, leading to ischaemic necrosis. The hernia becomes tender and swollen and the patient unwell. Symptoms and signs of intestinal obstruction are usually present, but may be absent in a Richter's hernia with strangulation of only part of the bowel wall, or if the hernia contains only omentum. The white-cell count is invariably raised. Treatment is resuscitation and analgesia followed by surgery to reduce the hernia, resection of any necrotic gut and repair of the hernial defect. General anaesthesia is usually preferred. Local anaesthetic may suffice for a low approach to the femoral canal, but bowel resection is difficult.

37. (a) F.
    (b) F.
    (c) T.
    (d) F.
    (e) T.

The decision of when to admit a patient is difficult and is often left to the most junior members of a team. However, the nature and severity of the injury, the general condition and social support of the patient have to be considered and it is not possible categorically to state that admission is not necessary purely on one factor. Loss of consciousness, skull fracture and vomiting are associated with increased risk of intracranial haematoma, but haematomas can be found on a CT scan after relatively minor injury. It is debatable whether it is necessary to remove these surgically.

Increased intracranial pressure causes damage to vital centres in the midbrain resulting in bradycardia and hypertension. These signs must be taken in context with other signs, including the level of consciousness (assessed using the Glasgow Coma Scale) and pupil size and response to light. Other signs that may be due to increased intracranial pressure include reduced respiratory rate and hyperpyrexia.

Depressed skull fractures, unless minor, are associated with an increased risk of epilepsy and are usually elevated.

If they overly a venous sinus, surgery is usually avoided because of the risk of bleeding. Leakage of cerebrospinal fluid from the nose (rhinorrhoea) or from the ear (otorrhoea) indicates that the dura mater has been torn and is often found after a fracture of the base of the skull. Antibiotics are given until the leak stops, which usually happens spontaneously, but occasionally requires surgical repair of the dura mater with a patch.

38. (a) T.
    (b) T.
    (c) F.
    (d) T.
    (e) F.

Over 80% of patients with bladder tumours have haematuria, but some do not. Sterile pyuria is also suggestive of a bladder tumour. If the patient has had long-term unnoticed haematuria they may present with a microcytic hypochromic anaemia. Treatment depends on the staging of the disease by cystoscopic appearance, biopsy and bimanual examination. Regular 'check cystoscopies' are required as recurrence is high, but responds to further treatment. Bladder tumours may respond to systemic chemotherapy, but local instillation of a chemotherapeutic agent into the bladder is particularly effective.

39. (a) F.
    (b) T.
    (c) F.
    (d) T.
    (e) T.

The aetiology of Menière's disease, consisting of tinitis, vertigo and neurosensory deafness, is unknown. It tends to be episodic with periods of remission, although after each attack hearing may decline. Stimulation of the labyrinth with cold water fails to produce the normal response of nystagmus. Acute attacks are controlled with promethazine and chlorpromazine. Long-term treatment of the condition is unsatisfactory.

40. (a) T.
    (b) F.
    (c) T.
    (d) T.
    (e) T.

Popliteal artery aneurysms are the second commonest peripheral artery aneurysm (aortic are the commonest) and the commonest presentation is due to embolization of thrombotic material into the distal circulation or thrombosis resulting in acute limb ischaemia. Rupture can occur but is unusual. Surgical salvage of the limb in the acute presentation can be difficult, as the small vessels in the calf may contain thrombus and streptokinase may be used to lyse this prior to surgical intervention.

The commonest surgical treatment is an exclusion bypass. This will be associated with a low failure rate, but can result in limb loss. As many of these patients are elderly it has been suggested that if a PAA is small and does not contain thrombus on ultrasound scan it can be observed safely.

41. (a) T.
    (b) T.
    (c) F.
    (d) T.
    (e) F.

Bunions (hallux valgus) are very common and due to increased prominence of the first metatarsal head associated with widening of the forefoot and lateral deviation of the proximal phalanx. They occur mainly in the elderly, but can be seen in teenagers, especially if there is a strong family history of bunions. The patient usually complains of pain and deformity. In young patients deformity may be the only complaint. Simple adjustment of footwear (wide-fitting shoes) is often sufficient to reduce the discomfort. In young patients the deformity is reduced by osteotomy of the first metatarsal. Commonly, excision of the prominent part of the metatarsal head (the proximal third of the proximal phalanx) allows a fibrous union to occur (Keller's procedure, which is an excision arthroplasty).

42. (a) F.
    (b) F.
    (c) T.
    (d) F.
    (e) T.

The natural history of asymptomatic aneurysms is unclear. Below 5 cm the risk of rupture is extremely small, at 5–6 cm probably 7–10% per year, but over 6 cm most accept that the risk of rupture is high (20–40% per year). With careful pre-operative assessment mortality from repair can be reduced to 2–5%, which is better than the mortality from rupture (estimated at 85%). Selection for surgery is based not on age but on the general state of the patient and the size of the aneurysm. Few patients develop symptoms in advance of rupture. A tender aneurysm is an indication for urgent intervention, but the operative mortality will be higher than for elective surgery, which is obviously preferential.

The aneurysm is not removed, but a bypass graft is inlaid into the sac, and sutured to non-aneurysmal artery above and below. The sac is then closed over the graft which separates it from other structures. After initial recovery very few patients develop late complications and so the outlook is excellent.

Less than 5% of aortic aneurysms extend above the renal arteries. These can be treated satisfactorily, although the operative risks are greater and this must be balanced against the general condition of the patient.

43. (a) F.
    (b) F.
    (c) T.
    (d) T.
    (e) T.

Rupture of the Achilles tendon tends to occur in middle age during sudden muscular exertion such as jumping. The patient often complains that it felt as if a blow was received from behind and the gap in the tendon may be felt. However, diagnosis can be difficult and the condition must be distinguished from tears of the calf muscles and deep vein thrombosis. With the patient prone, squeezing the calf will normally cause plantar flexion of the foot, but no movement will occur if the tendon is ruptured (Simmond's test).

Treatment involves immobilizing the tendon with the ends in close proximity by placing the foot in equinus in a plaster until healing has occurred. Alternatively, the ends of the tendon are sutured, but the patient still has to wear a plaster for 8 weeks. Which is the best treatment is controversial, and also depends on the general condition and expectations of the patient in terms of physical activity. It is claimed by some that surgical repair gives a better functional result.

44. (a) T.
    (b) T.
    (c) T.
    (d) F.
    (e) T.

Diverticula usually occur between the antimesenteric and mesenteric taeniae of the sigmoid colon due to the high intracolic pressures generated by a diet inadequate in fibre. 90% of cases remain asymptomatic, but complications include acute diverticulitis, which has been named 'left-sided appendicitis'. When signs are localized to the left iliac fossa, treatment is by intravenous fluids and antibiotics. A peridiverticular abscess may be drained percutaneously, but when acutely inflamed diverticula perforate, faecal peritonitis results. Laparotomy is required, with a thorough washout followed by excision of the diseased bowel and exteriorization of the descending colon (Hartmann's operation).

45. (a) T.
    (b) T.
    (c) F.
    (d) F.
    (e) F.

Lateral dislocation of the patella can occur, especially in young women, without obvious injury. Spontaneous reduction usually occurs. Rarely this is due to a congenital abnormality of the patella, but more often is said to be associated with an increased angle between the quadriceps and the patella due to widening of the pelvis at puberty or failure of normal development of the lower end of the femur. Following the first episode of dislocation the capsule on the medial side of the patella is torn, and if it fails to unite recurrent dislocation will occur. Lateral pressure on the patella may cause a feeling of imminent dislocation in the patient and be resisted (the apprehension test). Often the patella has spontaneously reduced by the time of presentation and treatment is splintage to allow the best chance of the capsule to heal. If dislocation becomes recurrent surgical intervention is required – either release of the lateral side of the joint capsule with plication of the medial side or medial relocation of the insertion of the patella tendon.

Chondromalacia patellae is a condition in which softening of the articular cartilage on the patella occurs. This results in fissuring and destruction of the cartilage, causing pain and discomfort. This tends to occur in young girls, and direct pressure on the patella during knee flexion may cause discomfort. Treatment is initially conservative, involving rest, anti-inflammatory drugs and analgesia. If the symptoms are severe and progressive, surgical intervention – either realignment of the patella or shaving the posterior surface – may be undertaken. The prognosis is good and most patients recover, but a few develop osteoarthritis.

Traction injury to the apophysis at the site of insertion of the patella tendon (Osgood–Schlatter's disease) may cause local pain and tenderness. Disruption of the apophysis can be seen on X-ray in some cases. Spontaneous recovery usually occurs.

Fracture of the patella occurs either due to a direct blow, in which case the bone is often shattered (stellate fracture), or by transmission of force through the extensor mechanism which can result in transverse fracture. As the patella is contained within the capsule of the knee, the bone fragments should be contained. In most cases the bone is allowed to unite and early movement is allowed to encourage moulding. If malunion occurs and causes problems, patellectomy can be undertaken. This is rarely undertaken in the first instance unless the fracture is severely comminuted. Displaced transverse fractures of the patella must be surgically reduced and fixed, otherwise knee extension will be reduced.

46. (a) T.
    (b) F.
    (c) F.
    (d) F.
    (e) T.

Epididymal cysts are common and often multiple. They occur behind the testicle in the epididymis or between it and the testicle. They do not cause infertility, but surgical removal can. Injection sclerotherapy is painful and not effective, and treatment is surgical removal. They are harmless and can be left in many cases.

47. (a) T.
    (b) F.
    (c) F.
    (d) T.
    (e) F.

True phimosis is a very tight foreskin, producing a pinhole meatus, with pain and ballooning of the prepuce on micturition. The treatment is circumcision. The foreskin (prepuce) is usually non-retractile until the age of 3–4 years, after which time *gentle* parental bathtime manipulation may be necessary to encourage full retraction. Forceful retraction at a younger age may cause tearing, resulting in balanitis and secondary phimosis, but parental education, not circumcision, is the treatment of a single episode of balanitis. In children, circumcision under local anaesthetic would be very frightening for the child and difficult for the surgeon. There is a reduced incidence of carcinoma of the penis in races that routinely circumcise for religious reasons.

48. (a) T.
    (b) F.
    (c) F.
    (d) T.
    (e) F.
    A generalized increase in vascular permeability occurs in all patients. In the lung the lymphatic system copes with this at first, but eventually becomes overwhelmed. There is evidence of some degree of pulmonary oedema in most patients and, if the attack is severe, may lead to respiratory failure. Although transient glycosuria may occur, insulin is rarely required and hypocalcaemia often occurs after 24–48 hours. Pseudocysts (collections in the lesser sac) occur in about 12% of patients and 50% resolve without intervention. There is no evidence that bacteria are implicated in uncomplicated acute pancreatitis, although secondary infection of necrotic tissue may occur.

49. (a) T.
    (b) F.
    (c) F.
    (d) T.
    (e) T.
    Foreign bodies lodged in the external canal may cause irritation and infection, resulting in discharge. This is more common in children. External otitis can be diffuse, and if chronic may produce a discharge. Uncomplicated acute otitis media and perforation of the ear drum do not result in discharge.
    Cholesteatoma is a complication of chronic suppurative otitis media. Part of the tympanic membrane becomes invaginated and the epithelial lining cells are trapped, enclosed in the invaginated part of the drum. They form a mass which continues to enlarge and causes local destruction. A chronic discharge occurs which often become secondarily infected.

50. (a) T.
    (b) F.

(c) F.
(d) T.
(e) F.

A false aneurysm sac does not include the three layers of the arterial wall, and commonly follows a penetrating injury to an artery such as a stab wound, needle or catheter puncture or arterial surgery. False aneurysms less commonly form after blunt injury. Initial bleeding results in a haematoma in the surrounding tissues. This may liquify and form a direct communication with the arterial lumen via the original injury. This can be difficult to distinguish from a simple haematoma, and duplex ultrasound will demonstrate the lumen of an aneurysm with blood flow in it.

Small false aneurysms will occasionally thrombose spontaneously and can be safely left. This can be encouraged by compression under ultrasound control. Most aneurysms remain patent and require treatment to avoid the risk of rupture, thrombosis of the aneurysm and underlying vessels or embolization. Treatment usually requires excision of the aneurysm sac with repair of the underlying vessel to avoid ischaemia. Some aneurysms will be infected, and in these cases a bypass graft may have to be routed around the infected area.

INDEX

Abdomen, acute, 4
Abdominal aortic aneurysms (AAA), 1, 62
Abdominal pain, 38
  atrial fibrillation with shock and, 56
Abdominal surgery
  diabetes in, 20
  pain relief after, 4
  wound infection after, 5
Accidents
  head injury in road traffic, 31
  motorcyclist, 50
Achalasia of oesophagus, 11
Achilles tendon, rupture of, 63
Acute abdomen, 4
Acute pancreatitis, 1
Adenocarcinoma
  kidney, 13
  oesophagus, 1
Adenomatous polyps, large bowel, 19
Anaesthesia
  epidural, 8
  local analgesic (anaesthetic) infiltration, 21
Anal carcinomas, 16
Anal fissure, 52
Anal fistula, 59
Angiography, lower limb, 57
Ankylosing spondylitis, 59
Antibiotic prophylaxis, large bowel surgery, 33
Antidiuretic hormone (ADH), 16
Aortic aneurysm repair, 61
Aortic dissection, acute, 36
Aortic valve replacement, 28
Appendicitis, 39
  diagnosis of, 11
Arm, transient weakness, 55

Arteriovenous fistulas, 9
Atheromatous occlusion of superficial femoral artery, 3
Atheromatous stenosis of renal artery, 14–15
Atrial fibrillation with shock and severe abdominal pain, 56
Atrial septal defect, 25
Aural discharge, 64
Axillary lymph nodes, breast cancer involving, 13

Basal cell carcinoma of the skin, 31
Bladder tumours, 60
  transitional cell, 61
Bleeding, *per rectum*, 57
Blood transfusion, 37
Bone
  metastatic carcinoma, 22
  secondary tumours, 53
Breast
  fibroadenomas, 15
  investigation of lump, 53–4
Breast cancer
  early, 44–5
  invasive ductal carcinoma, 41
  involving axillary lymph nodes, 13
  mammographic screening for, 2
Bunions, 62
Burns, 9, 42
  assessment, 33

Carcinomas
  characteristics of, 7–8
  see also specific type and specific organ
Carpal tunnel syndrome, 2–3
Cervical ribs, 45
Cervical spine, rheumatoid arthritis (RA), 10–11

INDEX

Chest drain, 29
Childbirth, urinary incontinence, 44
Cholecystitis, acute, 36
Circumcision, 64
Colles fracture, 7
Colon
  carcinoma of, 29–30
  diverticular disease of, 21, 63
Colorectal cancer, 49
  risk factors, 21
Congenital dislocation of the hip, 24
Coronary artery bypass grafting (CABG), 1
Crohn's disease, 28
Crush fractures, lumbar vertebrae, 9
Cyclical mastalgia, 19
Cyst. *See* Epididymal cyst; Sebacious cyst
Cystic hygroma, 58

Day-case surgery, 34
Deep vein thrombosis (DVT), 10, 15, 23, 27, 29
Diabetes in abdominal surgery, 20
Diverticular disease of the colon, 21, 63
Duodenal ulcers, 3
Dupuytren's contracture, 41

Ear, aural discharge, 64
Endoscopic retrograde cholangio-pancreatography (ERCP), 57
Epididymal cysts, 63
Epidural anaesthesia, 8
Epistaxis, 43

Fallot's tetralogy, 48
Familial adenomatous polyposis coli (FAP), 17
Femoral artery
  atheromatous occlusion, 3
  false aneurysm, 64
Femoral neck, fracture, 3, 6
Femoral shaft, fracture, 52
Femoropopliteal artery (below knee) bypass, 59–60
Fibroadenoma, breast, 15

Fistula, jejunum-abdominal skin, 36
Fistula-in-ano, 59
Fluid levels, 14
Fracture
  femoral shaft, 52
  humerus, 14, 48
  in children, 47
  mandible, 16
  neck of femur (NOF), 3, 6
  non-union, 44
  pelvis, 23
  proximal shaft of femur, 6
  radius, 48–9
  ribs, 10
  scaphoid bone, 43
  ulnar, 48–9
  wrist, 7
Fracture dislocation of spine, 10

Gallstone formation, 45
Ganglion, 27–8
Gas gangrene, 31
Glucocorticoid steroids, 46
Grave's disease, 27

Haematemesis, 60–1
Haematuria, 7
Haemorrhoids, 55, 56
Hand
  Raynaud's phenomenon, 36
  rheumatoid arthritis, 39
Head, trauma management, 61
Head injury in road traffic accident, 31
Hernia. *See* Hiatus hernia; Inguinal hernia; Strangulated femoral hernia
Hiatus hernia, paraoesophageal (rolling), 22
Hip
  congenital dislocation, 24
  osteoarthritis, 18
Hip pain, 24
Hirschsprung's disease, 13
Hoarseness of voice, 22
Hodgkin's disease, 49

INDEX

Humerus
  fracture, 14, 48
  supracondylar fracture, 14
Hydrocele, 30
Hydrocephalus, 4
Hyperparathyroidism, 45
Hypospadias, 28
Hypovalaemic shock, 27

Infantile hypertrophic pyloric stenosis, 35
Infrarenal aortic aneurysm repair, 34
Inguinal hernia, 3, 15, 51
Intermittent claudication, 3, 56
Internal carotid artery (ICA), 5
Intervertebral disc, prolapse of, 2
Intra-abdominal malignancy, 47
Intraperitoneal adhesions, 42
Intravenous fluid replacement, 17
Intussusception in children, 44
Irregular hepatomegaly, 53
Irritable bowel syndrome (IBS), 60
Ischaemia, leg amputation, 49–50
Ischaemic ulcers, 5

Jaundice
  management, 48
  obstructive, 29
Jejunum-abdominal skin fistula, 36

Kick in loin, 11
Kidney, adenocarcinoma of, 13
Knee
  medial meniscus of, 22–3
  pain investigation, 63
  sudden pain and tenderness, 30
Knee joint, osteoarthritis, 32

Laparoscopic cholecystectomy, 54
Large bowel, adenomatous polyps, 19
Large bowel surgery, antibiotic prophylaxis, 33
Larynx, tumours, 38
Leg
  acute ischaemia, 8–9
  oedema, 54

Leg amputation, ischaemia, 49–50
Limb. *See* Lower limb; Upper limb
Limp, 24
Lipoma, 16
Loin, kick in, 11
Lower limb
  angiography, 57
  ischaemic rest pain, 11
  venous ulcers, 51
Lumbar intervertebral disc, prolapse of, 28
Lumbar vertebrae, crush fractures, 9
Lung, squamous cell carcinoma, 6

Malaise, 53
Malignant melanoma, 4, 46
  prognosis, 9
Mammographic screening for breast cancer, 2
Mandible, fractures, 16
Maxillary antrum, carcinoma of, 18
Medial meniscus of knee, 22–3
Menière's disease, 62
Meningiomas, 54
Metastatic carcinoma in bone, 22

Nasal polyps, 33–4
Neck of femur (NOF), fractures, 3, 6
Necrotizing enterocolitis (NEC), new-born, 58
New-born
  failure to pass motion, 51
  necrotizing enterocolitis (NEC), 58
Nipple discharge, 24
Non-toxic nodular goitre (NTNG), 4

Obstructive jaundice, 29
Oesophagus
  achalasia, 11
  adenocarcinoma, 1
  atresia, 32
Osteoarthritis
  hip, 18
  knee joint, 32
Osteomyelitis, 55, 60

Osteosarcomas, 22
Ostium secundum, 25
Otitis media
  acute, 33
  secretory, 30

Pain relief after abdominal surgery, 4
Pancreas
  carcinoma, 14, 58
  carcinoma of head, 20
Pancreatitis
  acute, 1
  complications, 64
  management of severe acute, 7
Papillary carcinoma, thyroid, 9–10
Paraoesophageal (rolling) hiatus hernias, 22
Parotid region, palpable lump, 51
Pelvis, fracture, 23
Penis, carcinoma, 48
Peptic ulcer, perforated, 8
Perforated peptic ulcer, 8
Peripheral nerve (PN) injuries, 43
Peritonitis, symptoms and signs, 60
Phaeochromocytoma, 37, 50
Pharyngeal pouch, 44
Pharynx, tumours of, 5
Pituitary adenoma, 46
Pneumothorax, 20
Popliteal artery aneurysm (PAA), 62
Portal hypertension, 30
Portwine stains, 43
Prepatellar bursitis, 32–3
Primary thyrotoxicosis, 27
Prolapse of intervertebral disc, 2
Prolapse of lumbar intervertebral disc, 28
Prostate, carinoma of, 7
Prostate gland enlargement, 42
Prostatitis, 41
Proximal shaft of femur, fracture, 6
Pruritis ani, 58
Pulmonary embolism, post-operative, 46

Radius, fracture, 48–9
Raynaud's phenomenon, 36

Rectum, bleeding, 57
Reflux oesophagitis, 2
Renal artery, atheromatous stenosis of, 14–15
Renal stone, 18
Renal transplantation, 54
Rheumatoid arthritis, 56
  cervical spine, 10–11
  hand, 39
Rib
  cervical, 45
  fracture, 10
Road traffic accident, head injury in, 31

Salivary gland calculi, 59
Scaphoid bone, fracture, 43
Scoliosis of the spine, 8
Sebaceous cysts, 37
Secretory otitis media, 30
Seminoma of the testicle, 5
Septic shock syndrome, 23
Shoulder, dislocation, 12
Sigmoid volvulus, 47
Sinusitis, acute, 16
Skin
  basal cell carcinoma, 31
  portwine stains, 43
  squamous cell carcinoma, 52
Small bowel obstruction, 46
Sodium metabolism, 16
Spine
  fracture dislocation, 10
  scoliosis, 8
Splenectomy, 38
Squamous cell carcinoma
  lung, 6
  skin, 52
Stenosis of left internal carotid artery (ICA), 5
Stomach, carcinoma, 31–2, 34
Strangulated femoral hernia, 61
Strictures of urethra, 32
Stridor, 42
Subarachnoid haemorrhage (SAH), 6
Subdural empyema, 15

Superficial femoral artery, atheromatous occlusion, 3
Supracondylar fracture of the humerus, 14
Surgery, day-case, 34

Tennis elbow, 35
Testicle
  acutely painful, swollen, 53
  incompletely descended, 18
  seminoma, 5
  teratoma, 41
Thoracic outlet syndrome, 42
Thyroid, papillary carcinoma, 9–10
Thyroid nodule, 6
Tongue, cancer of, 14
Tonsillectomy, post-operative, 49
Tonsillitis, acute, 21
Total hip arthroplasty (THA), 19
Total parenteral nutrition, 57–8
Tracheo-oesophageal fistula (TOF), 32
Tracheostomy, 47
Transitional cell bladder tumours, 61
Tumour. *See* specific type and specific organ

Ulcer. *See* Duodenal ulcer; Ischaemic ulcer; Peptic ulcer; Venous ulcer

Ulcerative colitis (UC), 24
Ulnar, fracture, 48–9
Upper limb, surgical cervical (dorsal) sympathectomy, 37
Ureteric colic, 58–9
Ureteric stone, 2
Urethra, strictures of, 32
Urethral valves, posterior, 55
Urinary incontinence in childbirth, 44
Urinary retention, 35
Urine, vesicoureteric reflux of, 13

Varicose veins, 17, 19–20
Venous ulcers, 18, 50
  lower limb, 51
Vesicoureteric reflux of urine, 13
Voice, hoarseness of, 22
Vomiting, 29

Water control, 16
Weight loss, 53
Wound healing, 45
Wound infection after abdominal surgery, 5
Wrist
  Colles fracture, 7
  laceration, 37–8

SUBJECT AREAS

Paper and Question numbers given.

Anaesthetics
  Paper 1: 15, 35.
  Paper 2: 35.

Breast
  Paper 1: 8.
  Paper 2: 3, 13, 27, 49.
  Paper 4: 1, 18.
  Paper 5: 4.

Cardiothoracic
  Paper 1: 3, 26, 44.
  Paper 2: 7, 16, 22, 34, 39.
  Paper 3: 5, 10, 37.

Endocrine
  Paper 1: 14, 24, 41.
  Paper 3: 3, 43.
  Paper 4: 22, 42.

INDEX

Gastrointestinal
  Paper 1: 2, 5, 11, 18, 34, 47, 49.
  Paper 2: 15, 21, 28, 36, 37, 47.
  Paper 3: 6, 13, 21, 30, 40, 47, 48.
  Paper 4: 14, 27, 29, 39, 50.
  Paper 5: 10, 13, 15, 17, 23, 27, 30, 34, 44.

Hepatobiliary
  Paper 1: 4, 29.
  Paper 2: 5, 31.
  Paper 3: 9, 15, 38.
  Paper 4: 19, 32.
  Paper 5: 5, 18, 24, 48.

Metabolic
  Paper 1: 37.
  Paper 2: 8, 19, 33.
  Paper 3: 11, 27.
  Paper 4: 6, 25.
  Paper 5: 20.

Miscellaneous
  Paper 1: 13, 22, 42.
  Paper 2: 10, 18, 43.
  Paper 3: 2, 20, 28, 32, 42.
  Paper 4: 5, 21, 46.
  Paper 5: 8, 33, 36.

Neurosurgery
  Paper 1: 17, 25.
  Paper 2: 11.
  Paper 3: 7, 18.
  Paper 4: 23.
  Paper 5: 6, 37.

Oncology
  Paper 1: 19, 32.
  Paper 2: 38.
  Paper 4: 4, 30, 37.
  Paper 5: 1.

Otolaryngology
  Paper 1: 20.
  Paper 2: 7, 16, 22, 34, 39.
  Paper 3: 16, 26, 29, 46.
  Paper 4: 7, 11, 31, 38, 47.
  Paper 5: 21, 28, 39, 49.

Orthopaedics
  Paper 1: 6, 9, 10, 27, 31, 33, 39, 43, 45, 50.
  Paper 2: 6, 14, 24, 29, 40, 42, 46, 48.
  Paper 3: 17, 22, 25, 34, 45, 49.
  Paper 4: 3, 10, 13, 15, 28, 35, 36, 41.
  Paper 5: 3, 11, 16, 26, 32, 41, 43, 45.

Paediatric surgery
  Paper 2: 2, 4, 12, 26, 50.
  Paper 3: 8, 24, 36, 50.
  Paper 4: 17, 33, 44.
  Paper 5: 12, 22, 47.

Skin
  Paper 1: 16, 40.
  Paper 2: 17.
  Paper 3: 4, 19, 44.
  Paper 4: 12, 24, 49.

Urology
  Paper 1: 7, 28, 30, 46.
  Paper 2: 1, 25, 45.
  Paper 3: 14, 23, 33, 35.
  Paper 4: 2, 9, 16, 34.
  Paper 5: 2, 25, 31, 38, 46.

Vascular
  Paper 1: 1, 12, 21, 23, 36, 38, 48.
  Paper 2: 9, 20, 23, 30, 44.
  Paper 3: 1, 12, 31, 39, 41.
  Paper 4: 8, 20, 26, 40, 43, 45, 48.
  Paper 5: 7, 9, 14, 19, 29, 35, 40, 42, 50.